BEYOND REASON?

The first Stirling Professions and Management Conference was held in August 1993. Over 100 participants were drawn from the UK, Europe, Australasia and the USA and 75 papers were presented.

The main theme of the conference was the character of late twentieth century UK management, with a strong emphasis on the changing situations of professionals who have long been the bulk of the UK's managers. Over 30 of the conference papers are being published in three co-edited books as part of Avebury's Stirling Management Series. *The Professional-Managerial Class* (edited by Ian Glover and Michael Hughes) deals with the more general aspects of the main theme. *Professions at Bay* (same editors) focuses on the situations of over ten professions as they face the processes of managerialism, commercialism and consumerism. *Beyond Reason: the National Health Service and the Limits of Management* (edited by John Leopold, Ian Glover and Michael Hughes) is effectively a sector case study of the main themes. It asks whether 'science plus will' in the form of managerialism, allied to commercialism and consumerism are likely to make the National Health Service more effective, or debilitate it.

For Margaret, Cara and Euan

Beyond Reason?

The National Health Service and the limits of management

Edited by

JOHN LEOPOLD
IAN GLOVER
MICHAEL HUGHES
Department of Management and Organization
School of Management
University of Stirling

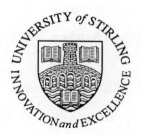

Avebury

Aldershot · Brookfield USA · Hong Kong · Singapore · Sydney

Published by
Avebury
Ashgate Publishing Ltd
Gower House
Croft Road
Aldershot
Hants GU11 3HR
England

Ashgate Publishing Company
Old Post Road
Brookfield
Vermont 05036
USA

British Library Cataloguing in Publication Data

Beyond Reason? National Health Service
        and the Limits of Management. - (Stirling
        Management Series)
        I. Leopold, John W.   II. Series
        362.1068

Library of Congress Catalog Card Number: 95-81147

ISBN 1 85972 031 5

Printed and bound by Athenaeum Press, Ltd.,
Gateshead, Tyne & Wear.

Contents

Figures and tables

List of contributors

Lynn Ashburner is a lecturer in Health Services Management at the University of Nottingham. She has published in the areas of gender, work organization, NHS and public sector management. Her current research interests include work organization and the health service professions.

Chris Bennett is a Senior Research Fellow at the Centre for Corporate Strategy and Change, University of Warwick. Much of her recent work has involved looking at different aspects of change within the NHS and other public sector bodies. She is co-author with Ewan Ferlie of *Managing Crisis and Change in Healthcare: the organizational response to HIV/AIDS* (Open University Press, 1994).

Colin Bryson was a Research Fellow in the Department of Management and Organization at the University of Stirling and has recently become a Teaching Research Fellow in the Department of Management at the University of St Andrews.

Sandra Dawson was Professor of Organizational Behaviour at Imperial College and in October 1995, Professor Dawson became the Peat Marwick Professor of Management Studies and Director of the Judge Institute of Management Studies at the University of Cambridge. Her present research interests focus on the Management of Professional Specialists, including medical doctors and lawyers as well as engineers and scientists. Professor Dawson is author of numerous articles and three books.

Sue Dopson is University Lecturer in Management Studies, Oxford University and Fellow in Organizational Behaviour at Templeton College. Her research interests span middle management work, exploring the relationship between R&D and clinical practice and health care management.

Louise FitzGerald is a Senior Lecturer at Warwick Business School, University of Warwick. Her research interests focus on the management of organizational change and current research is mainly in healthcare. She has published on processes of organizational change and the impact of change on professionals.

Ian Glover is a Lecturer in the Department of Management & Organization at the University of Stirling. His main research interests are managerial work and occupations in the UK and abroad.

Sheila Greenfield is Lecturer in Medical Sociology in the Department of General Practice and Research Fellow in the Department of Accounting & Finance at the University of Birmingham. She has published on topics in finance and management in General Practice, the training and organization of the primary health care team and the role of management information in small and large organizations.

James Harrison is a doctoral student at Aston Business School. He has research and publishing experience in health policy and management; current interests include corporate governance programme evaluation and marketing.

Michael Hughes is Professor, Deputy Head of the School of Management, and Head of the Department of Management & Organization at the University of Stirling. He is co-editor of *Rethinking Organization* (Sage, 1992).

Michael Jackson is Deputy Principal and Professor of Human Resources Management in the Department of Management & Organization at University of Stirling. He is author of *Policy Making in Trade Unions* (Avebury, 1991).

Michael Kelly is Professor and Head of School of Social Sciences at the University of Greenwich. He is a Medical Sociologist who has carried out work on the effects of chronic illness and preventing coronary heart disease. He has also worked on the Sociology of the Professions. His recent books include *Colitis* (Routledge, 1992) and *Healthy Cities* (Routledge, 1992).

John Leopold is Senior Lecturer in Human Resources Management at the University of Stirling. He has published a number of articles on industrial relations in the NHS, and is co-author of *The Decentralization of Collective Bargaining: An Analysis of Recent Experience in the UK* (Macmillan, 1993).

Terry McNulty is Senior Research Fellow at the Centre for Corporate Strategy and Change in Warwick Business School. He has published on organization and management issues in professional service organizations as well as the behaviour of boards and directors in large UK PLCs.

Veronica Mole is a Research Associate at The Management School, Imperial College of Science, Technology & Medicine. Her current research is on the strategic management of technology.

Amanda Nayak is a Lecturer in Accounting in the Department of Accounting & Finance at the University of Birminham. She has eight years professional and industrial accounting experience and has also lectured at Leicester Polytechnic and Massey University, New Zealand. Her research interests are appropriate accounting information for small businesses and finance and management in primary health care.

Sandra Nutley is a Lecturer in Management at the University of St Andrews. Her current research interests include: public sector management, organizational change, and the professions and management. She is co-author of *The Public Sector Management Handbook* (Longmans, 1994).

Jim Sherval was a research assistant at The Management School at Imperial College and is now a Researcher at the Centre for HIV/AIDS and Drug Studies of Lothian Health Board.

Ian Tilley is a Reader in Health Policy and Finance, Business School, University of Greenwich and Director of the University's NHS Organizational Change Project. He has published chiefly in the areas of finance and health management, including editing *Managing the internal market* (Paul Chapman, 1993).

Richard Whipp is Professor of Human Resource Management at, and Deputy Director of Cardiff Business School of the University of Wales. His main research interests are strategic change and the institutional analysis of sectors.

Richard Whittington is Senior Lecturer in Marketing and Strategic Management at Warwick Business School. He has published widely on strategic choice and change, and is author of two books, *Corporate Strategies in Recession and Recovery* (Unwin Hyman, 1989) and *What is Strategy-And Does It Matter?* (Routledge, 1993).

Acknowledgements

This book arose out of the first Stirling conference on Professions and Management in 1993. We are grateful to all the participants in that conference who helped shape the debate and the content of all three books in this series. In particular we would like to thank Mike Kelly of the University of Greenwich, a long time collaborator with Ian Glover, whose ideas helped structure and organize this book.

Sarah Anthony at Avebury was a very understanding editor who always managed to solve our technical problems.

Above all we are indebted to the tremendous skill and dedication of Terry Middleton who had the job of shaping thirteen chapters into the Avebury way. Not only did she have to coordinate the work of all the chapter authors, but she also had to get the three editors to work together and meet deadlines. In this she succeeded admirably.

Abbreviations

APAP	Association of Professional Ambulance Personnel
BMA	British Medical Association
BMJ	British Medical Journal
CCSC	Centre for Corporate Strategy and Change
CEO	Chief Executive Officer
CHC	Community Health Council
CCT	Compulsory Competitive Tendering
COHSE	Confederation of Health Service Employees
DoE	Department of Environment
DoH	Department of Health
DHSS	Department of Health and Social Security
DGH	District General Hospital
DHA	District Health Authorities
DMU	Directly Managed Unit
DPH	Director of Public Health
FHSA	Family Health Service Authority
FCE	Finished Consultant Episode
GMSC	General Medical Services Committee
GP	General Practitioner
GPFH	General Practitioner Fund Holder
GNP	Gross National Product
HA	Health Authority
HSSB	Health Services Supervisory Board
HRM	Human Resource Management
IRS	Industrial Relations Services

IPM	Institute of Personnel Management
LIG	London Implementation Group
MBA	Master of Business Administration
MOH	Medical Officer of Health
NAO	National Audit Office
NED	Non Executive Director
NHS	National Health Service
NHSME	National Health Service Management Executive
NHSTD	National Health Service Training Directorate
NHST	National Health Service Trust
PAM	Professions Allied to Medicine
PHM	Public Health Medicine
PHP	Public Health Physician
RHA	Regional Health Authorities
R&D	Research and Development
RAWP	Resource Allocation Working Party
RCM	Royal College of Midwives
RCN	Royal College of Nursing
SIFTR	Service Increment for Teaching and Research
TUC	Trades Union Congress
UGM	Unit General Managers
WfP	Working for Patients

Part I

INTRODUCTION AND CONTEXT

1 Introduction: Reason, rationality and the NHS

John Leopold, Ian Glover and Michael Hughes

This book has its origins in the first Professions and Management conference held at the University of Stirling in August 1993. The main theme of the conference was to explore the relationship between management and professionalism. Nowhere was that tension more apparent than in the National Health Service. A number of papers which sought to explore it are the basis of this book.

There is a long-standing debate about the significance and role of the general manager as opposed to the specialised professional. Some argue that 'management' is itself a profession with its own collection of practices and techniques which can be taught to aspirant 'professional managers'. The apotheosis of this view is the American MBA. By contrast, Sorge (1978) and Glover (1995) have praised the German approach based on the product of a very broad secondary education and then being broadly educated and trained in higher education in a vocational specialism first, whether this be as an engineer or as a commercial and financial specialist. These broadly educated specialists go on to form what English speakers call management, but in Germany the concept of 'general management' and indeed that of management itself, is eschewed and often derided. These themes and issues recur throughout this book. Can clinicians be developed into general managers, or is the introduction of general managers into the NHS needed because they can't, at least not in sufficient numbers?

To explore these issues Kelly and Glover present an overview of the attempts to organise and reorganise the delivery and management of health care in the United Kingdom since the creation of the NHS in 1948. Above all Kelly and Glover emphasise their view that there is a single line of evolution in the development of health care in Britain and that rhetoric used at each successive reorganisation to emphasise change, has in fact been designed, whether deliberately or not, to conceal continuity. The continuities, or single line of evolution, are based on the principles of rationality, efficiency and achievable good health for all. In effect they see all attempts to reorganise the NHS as being based on the modernist project of liberating humanity through providing health for all and achieving this by using scientific rationality to solve problems of human morbidity and organizational inefficiency in the NHS. Kelly and Glover regard these two concerns as fallacies; neither excellent health for all, nor the highly efficient management of the NHS is seen as being readily achievable.

Thus, in contrast to some other commentators, they stress the continuity of reorganizations; all have been designed to manage the delivery of health care services through some kind of organizational framework. While many commentators concur with this view with regard to the establishment of the NHS and the 1994 reorganization, Glover and Kelly argue that this was also true of Thatcher inspired changes such as the Griffiths' general management of 1983 and the consumerism of *Promoting Better Health* and *Working for Patients*. While administrative, then bureaucratic and finally market-driven concerns may have characterised successive reforms, underlying each reorganisation was the modernist belief that *an* answer existed to the problems confronting the NHS.

Kelly and Glover attempt to relate these developments in health care management to the role of administrative-professional thought in British management and the dominance of professions, especially that of doctors in the management of health care. These themes are explored in greater depth in the concluding chapter.

Underpinning Kelly and Glover's arguments about the health service is the argument found in Crook et al. (1992, p. 10) that differentiation, commodification and rationalization 'define the transformation of premodern into modern systems as well as the central processes of modern societies'. Modernization leads to a society that is highly differentiated, with high levels of specialization and complexity, and highly organized with high levels of rationalization and commodification. Moreover, for Crook et al. (1990, p. 32) 'postmodernization may be analysed as the consequence of the extension of the two modernization processes to extreme levels.' Hence hyper-differentiation, hyper-rationalization and hyper-commodification.

Kelly and Glover analyse the attempts to reorganize the NHS as standing for the grand narrative of modernism. Commodification, differentiation and rationalization are used to structure what follows in this book. Following the introduction and context, Part Two is based on the commodification of health, on attempts to introduce markets and exchange relations into health; Part Three on the differentiation of health care and its associated specializations e.g. acute and community, professions and administration, teaching and general hospitals; while Part Four is based on rationalization, on attempts to develop and control an efficiently managed legal-rational bureaucratic structure.

Commodification

In Chapter Three Bryson, Jackson and Leopold examine the role of human resource managers as initiators and influencers of change in NHS trusts. Of particular importance here is their role as 'conformist innovators' who identify with the objective of organizational success, but conform to the criteria governing the means of its achievement adopted by managerial colleagues, who usually have greater power than they have. The dilemma for NHS human resource managers is that there are two competing groups of managerial colleagues; the potential conflict between 'professional management' and 'general management' as identified by Kelly and Glover. Therefore human resource directors who sought to adopt a 'conformist innovator' model would need to be clear about which was the dominant coalition in the trust to align themselves with.

The challenge for NHS trust human resource directors was to bring about change in pay determination; to move away from the highly centralised, highly prescribed bargaining in Whitley Councils and national determination through Pay Review Bodies, to more decentralised methods which may include local bargaining and more managerially decided pay determination for some groups of staff. At the time of the research on which this chapter is based little change had been effected despite support for change from the government and many senior NHS managers.

Harrison et al. (1992, p. 100) argue that 'general management has not even challenged the medical domain never mind having succeeded in making significant in roads into it', although they concede that it has increased the authority of managers over other professionals. From the viewpoint of human resource managers this underscores their dilemma. If they are to ally with general managers, then their attempts at change may be thwarted by the power of professional groups, especially doctors. If they seek alliances with doctors, they may find their approaches rebuffed as doctors are powerful enough to resist unwelcome change at the local level. Evidence of the ambiguous position of human resource managers is presented which suggests that the 'conformist innovator' approach only exists in a limited number of cases and that the dominant form of personnel management in NHS trusts remains, as pre-trust, the 'contracts manager', subordinate to both managerialism and professionalism.

The drive to bring a market orientation to bear in health care delivery has also affected general practitioners. New contracts for general practitioners were introduced in 1990 which aimed to make general practices more business like. From 1991 onwards budget holding was introduced; general practitioners were forced to take on a management role. In Chapter Four Greenfield and Nayak examine the responses of a sample of general practitioners to these changes.

A key finding was the general hostility of general practitioners to having a management role thrust upon them. The responses demonstrate a clear tension between the professional role of a doctor and the alien role of a manager. The respondents' comments indicate the disdain that professional doctors have for managers, management, commerce and accountants.

5

Greenfield and Nayak also tried to assess how general practitioners were coping with the new contract after one year of operation. They concluded that doctors are struggling with the new situation, but surprisingly only just over one third expressed a need for training. Muddling through seemed to be the order of the day. General practitioners had not taken to management.

In the final chapter in this section McNulty, Whittington and Whipp explore the work experiences of doctors, scientists and engineers as they become subject to market control through the internal market of the NHS or the market control of industrial R&D. They regard the conceptual approach offered by the sociology of professions as inadequate for studying the relations between work and markets. It is seen as concentrating on the organization of professions and an occupational level of analysis rather than the work activity and an individual level of analysis. Thus they emphasise the need to concentrate on what actually happens in the workplace, rather than away from it, in order to understand professional and managerial work. They therefore draw upon Macintyre (1990) and Keat (1991) and focus on the concept of 'practice' to focus on the practices of medicine, engineering and science. They expect that the pressures on doctors, scientists and engineers will intensify as NHS hospitals and industrial R&D labs are subjected to greater market control. Consequently these practitioners are likely to experience conflict in relationships with both the market and the organization that they work in.

From their analysis of the work of 158 doctors, scientists or engineers working in four NHS hospitals and four industrial R&D laboratories, McNulty et al. find support for the view that practices are vulnerable to market control. They present evidence that internal goods and practice standards of excellence can be undermined by reduced funding for long-term medical and scientific research, as well as other negative features.

However, they also found that in some cases market forces can enhance practice standards of excellence and offer different opportunities for practitioners to realise internal goods. These dual findings suggest that the arguments of Macintyre (1990) and Keat (1991) are too one dimensional and that the two-way direction of impact put forward in their model captures the situation better. McNulty et al. therefore call for further research to examine under what conditions practices are vulnerable or enhanced.

Differentiation

A feature of the development of medicine has been its increased specialisation. Since 1948 this differentiation of health care has been manifested in a number of ways; in the difference between acute and community care, between teaching and general hospitals, between different medicine specialisms, between clinical and non-clinical specialists. This theme of differentiation is addressed in Part Three.

Medicine is differentiated in the hierarchy of grades, but also between specialities so that there is both conflict and consensus, and isolationism and cooperation, within and between these specialities. In Chapter Six Bennett addresses the response of medical professionals to HIV/AIDS within the specific organizational context of the medical speciality. All the medical specialities most closely involved with the HIV/AIDS issue were, to some extent 'Cinderella specialists' within the health service hierarchy and therefore unlikely candidates to make a major impact on service delivery. Bennett analyses the way in which, despite this disadvantage, medical professionals from these specialities played key roles in the development of the response to HIV/AIDS.

She analyzes this contribution during three 'stages'; a pre-legitimation stage (1981-1986); a legitimation stage (1986-1987); and a post legitimation stage (1987 onwards). She argues that the success of key medical professionals was due to the combination of the archetypical characteristics of professionals (status, autonomy, collegiality) with the characteristics of entrepreneurs (single-mindedness, drive, enthusiasm). Thus we have the emergence of clinical 'product champions' who through their individual characteristics were able to overcome the disadvantage of the low status of their speciality. But in the case of HIV/AIDS the development of expertise was done in collaboration with patients and voluntary sector social movement organizations. This, it is argued, was not a total transfer of professional power to consumer interests, but a process of 'giving away' power in one direction, in order to keep it by remaining the focus of service provision.

Bennett identifies a drop in interest in HIV/AIDS after 1990 and suggests that the expansion of appointments as HIV professionals in health authorities meant that many of these post holders are working in authorities where there is no powerful medical product champion for the issue and therefore are not able to affect service development in the way in which the pioneers of the cause were. Bennett raises interesting questions for future research about the extent to which those medical specialists who gained status in the first two stages are able to sustain these gains in the third, or do they need to champion new causes in order to sustain their new position in the differentiation of the medical specialisms?

Two types of differentiation are addressed by Tilley in Chapter Seven. First it is a study of acute hospitals, but more importantly it focuses on the inter and intra professional relations involved in recent changes in policy affecting the inner London teaching hospital. These include the general post 1990 reforms, as well as more specific reviews affecting health care in London.

Central to Tilley's argument is the concept of disjunctions, or a mis-match between contracts and resources. Four types of disjunctions are identified. These are L1, where workloads actually achieved vary from the contract; L2, where beds allocated and/or clinical staff numbers do not respond to contracts; L3, where the budget allocation does not adjust to the contract; and L4, where the speciality under or overspends its budget allocation. These disjunctions are seen as the outcomes of power and influence within the 'politically negotiated order' (Bacharach and Lawler, 1980) of the interest groups in and outside the hospital, but focusing on the position of the differentiated specialities within the acute hospital. The main source of data is two London teaching hospitals.

While recognising that the analysis presented is a preliminary one, Tilley identifies continuing, indeed increasing disjunctions of all four types. Specialism 'winners' (oncology, renal) and 'losers' (surgery, psychiatry) are identified. Intra-professional power relations between the specialisms are seen to be of more importance in determining these outcomes than inter-professional relations between doctors and other health care workers.

In the differentiation of medical specialities there are higher and lower status specialisms. In Chapter Eight Dawson, Sherval and Mole examine the changing position of Public Health Physicians, a group of doctors who have traditionally been regarded as being of low status and influence, but who under the recent reforms, now have an opportunity to relocate their position in both the medical and managerial hierarchies. But as the title of the chapter suggests, in so doing Public Health Physicians have to resolve the dilemma of whether they are in or out of management.

In a useful summary of the historical position of the public health profession, Dawson, Sherval and Mole demonstrate that it has been one of uncertainty and low morale and status. This uncertainty is perhaps reflected in the changing job title attached to its practitioners; Medical Office of Health, Community Medicine and now Public Health Medicine. From the establishment of the NHS in 1948, each reorganisation left them on the margins as the preoccupations of more ascendant groups were to the fore.

However, the introduction of the purchaser/provider split with its emphasis on addressing the health needs of the country rather than the interests of the providing institutions, creates an opportunity for Public Health Physicians to provide advice and information about health care needs which can potentially influence the purchasing decision in a major way. This then has the potential to alter the status position of Public Health Physicians vis a vis other medical specialists, allowing them to become part of strategic managerial process of purchasing, but which may challenge their traditional position of 'independence'. Hence the 'in or out of management' dilemma.

Dawson, Sherval and Mole draw upon their empirical research in ten provider organizations to examine these issues. In the context of this volume a major finding is reaffirmation of the view expressed in much of the literature that there is an uncertain relationship between public health doctors and management, perhaps summed up by one respondent who felt that there was an 'appalling ignorance of management and of health by both areas'. The central dilemma of the chapter remains unresolved, and so too is the question of whether Public Health Physicians will be able to seize the opportunity presented by their potentially strategic position in health care purchasing to re-establish themselves as key strategic players in the differentiated hierarchy of medicine.

The relationship between doctors and management is explored further by Dopson in Chapter Nine. She begins by reviewing the evidence from various ethnographic studies of health care systems on the nature of doctors' involvement in management of health services. She finds an unwillingness of doctors to be involved in local, as opposed to national, management, but attributes this to their considerable influence as doctors without therefore a need to adopt a formal management role. While one of the thrusts of the Griffiths Report was to curtail the power of the medical profession through the introduction of general management, the review of the literature presented here suggests that this has not happened.

Dopson, following Fleck (1979), relates the reluctance of doctors to be involved in management to the differences in thought styles between doctors and managers which suggests that there is a fundamental conflict of interests at the social structural level. Despite this, since the introduction of the internal market into the NHS, there have been continuing attempts to involve doctors in management; attempts synthesised by Hunter (1991) into the creation of the doctor-manager, the consultant as clinical director.

Dopson's empirical work is based on interviews with hospital consultants undergoing a training programme for potential clinical directors. The continuing reluctance of consultants to become involved in management and their relationship to management was summed up by one consultant who said 'management is the one disease I did not think existed'. They became involved in management to stop non-consultants managing them, and had a poor opinion of managers in the NHS. While negative views predominated, some respondents saw involvement in management as a positive way to increase their power base. Dopson explores the tensions and ambiguities associated with attempts to create the doctor-manager.

Issues concerning the adoption of management roles by clinicians are developed further in Chapter Ten. Drawing on a small sample of thirty one clinicians who had assumed management roles in a health care provider unit, FitzGerald examines how the changes in health care management impact on individual clinicians and the way the changes affect intra-professional boundaries and on the interfaces between doctors and managers. In particular she addresses whether or not the medical profession continues in its position of dominance and suggests that UK doctors, like their US counterparts, are able to maintain this through adapting to circumstances (Freidson, 1987).

In contrast to Dopson's finding in the previous chapter, FitzGerald's cohort had a positive view of their management role and wanted to influence the direction or form of change, and, indeed, could see ways of doing this. FitzGerald argues that since Griffiths in 1983, a combination of environmental, organisational, and individual factors have altered clinicians' past judgements about management and about their role within it. In summary, the creation of the purchase/provider split, the part-time nature of the clinical director post, and the personal challenge of the role, acting in combination have led to a reassessment of the relationship between doctors and management. She presents some initial evidence from a second, related, study on the significant impact of clinical directors on trust boards. Interestingly in terms of the dilemmas discussed in Chapter Eight, she suggests that some Medical Directors and Directors of Public Health have considerable influence because they act as 'licensed dissenters'.

FitzGerald does identify some negative aspects to the role of clinical managers which is more supportive of Dopson's evidence. Given that both these studies were based on small samples and conducted in the early years of operation of the new system, there is clearly a need for continued research into these issues.

FitzGerald also addresses the question of inter and intra professional relationships. Although her cohort was unusual in that they all had prior management training, their perceptions of management were relatively unsophisticated and largely centred on 'people' skills. The training programme they undertook widened these perceptions considerably especially in terms of understanding strategic management, marketing and business policy. This, it is suggested, altered both their relationships with non-clinical managers and their ability to influence decisions.

In terms of relationships with medical colleagues, there was some evidence that issues of professional performance and professional standards were being addressed by clinical managers in a way that had been avoided by General Managers. This, and other factors, meant that relationships with medical colleagues could be difficult at times, leading to isolation. Potentially, some clinical managers could be rejected by the rest of the medical profession, but not accepted by managers. A further challenge to the traditional collegiality of the medical profession may come in the competition between NHS trusts for contracts and resources.

Rationalization

The issues raised by the process of differentiation in the NHS have been explored in some depth in Chapters Six to Ten. We now turn to examine the importance of rationalization. In Part Four we address issues concerning the legal-rational bureaucratic structure of the state and its role in funding, managing and directing the NHS. Various reorganisations of the NHS have been attempts to rationalize its structure and epitomise the centralising tendencies of the state. The post 1990 reforms are often seen as a shift of one type of rationality, managerialism, which characterised the NHS from 1948-1990, to a new rationality, consumerism. While some commentators have stressed the discontinuity between these stages, the underlying theme of this book is the continuing view that all the reforms are based on the premise that a rational system of organization is possible whether it is based on managerialism or consumerism. Moreover, managerialism as aggressively directed at professions, with the latters' disdain for the commercial, *would* be expected to manifest itself, in some respects, as consumerism.

Ashburner, in Chapter Eleven, addresses the relationship between professions and managerialism, and in so doing raises questions about the traditional concept of a profession. She suggests that the context of NHS restructuring in the 1990s and the challenge of professional management is different from the past and might, therefore, made the traditional process of the medical profession establishing and defending its boundaries more difficult.

As the writers of chapters discussed previously have pointed out, the medical profession in the UK had remained dominant over other health professions and has successfully adapted to change. In particular it had resisted the Griffiths' attempt to bring doctors into management. Cox (1991) saw this attempt at rationalization as inappropriate because the NHS did not resemble a bureaucracy but a loosely structured order.

Drawing upon data collected by a variety of means over a three year period, Ashburner examines the impact of the purchaser/provider split, GP fund holding and the role of the newly constituted health authorities and trusts. The work is based on the view that a combination of the number of reforms, their ideological nature and the persistence of government focus means that this situation is different from past attempts at reform both in the processes and the direction in which they are moving.

If managerialism is on the rise in the NHS, then this may pose a threat to the key concepts of medical autonomy and medical dominance. The maintenance of clinical autonomy is seen as key to professional power in the NHS, although the relative importance of this is debated. Ashburner concludes that doctors have been able to respond to the external changes by a process of adaptation so as to maintain their autonomy and power. For example, the part-time nature of clinical director posts means that clinicians can be involved in management without having to give up clinical practice. However, as Dopson argued in Chapter Nine, this may mean that clinical directors are seen as not being a full part of either the medical profession or of management.

Ashburner does, however, argue that professionalization and bureaucratization should not be seen as opposing forces. Not only is accommodation possible but the two groups can even work well together. Her evidence suggests that management and doctors can cooperate without affecting clinical autonomy, and indeed, that they can have shared values. In short, she calls for further exploration of the concept of managerialism and professionalism as companion, rather than opposing, processes. In particular she suggests that managers and professionals may have shared objectives in dealing with pressures from outside the unit.

This research also has implications for the differentiation debate as it probes shifts in the balance of power between hospital doctors, GP fund holders and Public Health Physicians. For example, GP fund holders now find that hospital clinicians relate to them in a different way because of their ability to move patients in a number of directions and the rising status of Public Health Physicians discussed in Chapter Eight is confirmed.

However Ashburner's research does indicate contradictory tendencies; not all clinicians welcome a management role. GPs have to work out an appropriate relationship with practice managers, and not all Public Health Physicians welcome the loss of their 'independent' role. The continuing lack of homogeneity in the profession may suggest limits to the medical profession's ability to resist changes that might impinge on their autonomy, but Ashburner concludes that adaptation, partly on doctors own terms, would appear to be more protective of their position in the long term.

In the final chapter in this section Harrison and Nutley further examine the relationship between professions and management, by offering a comparison between the NHS and local government. In the context of our theme about rationalization of the public sector they examine recent strategies for introducing managerialism into the public sector; a form of managerialism that stresses rationality and calculation which undermine more abstract notions of 'service' or 'the public good' (Morgan, 1990).

Harrison and Nutley also caution us not to regard the relationship between professionals and management as being solely a conflictual one. Indeed, drawing from Morgan (1990), it is stressed that the professional commitment to expertise makes wholesale opposition to rationalization impossible.

In their health service example, they see the introduction of general management following the Griffiths Report and the implementation of *Working for Patients* (DHSS, 1989) as the two most important strategies used by the government to introduce managerialism to the NHS. This perhaps gives a different weight to the view expressed in earlier chapters that general management did not alter the power and status of the medical profession fundamentally. But in reviewing their case study District Health Authority they argue both that general management challenged and weakened professional authority in various ways, and that it had only limited success in harnessing and directing the more senior profession of medicine. This latter point confirms the findings presented in Part Three.

Local government has also been subjected to a barrage of legalization and reforms under the post 1979 Conservative governments, and individual authorities have also sought to change their ways of operating. Departmentalism gave way to corporatism, which in turn gave way to consumerism and decentralization. All the reforms can be seen as a direct challenge to local government professionalism.

Harrison and Nutley are unwilling to characterise the conflicts within their case study local authority as conflict between professionalism and managerialism. Departmentalism and inter professional conflict were more to the fore than a simple professionalism versus managerialism kind of conflict. Indeed departmental managers used the rhetoric of the new managerialism to defend their departmental interests against others without fully embracing it.

They also explore the political domain as it affects both these sectors. Following Stewart and Walsh (1992) they see an attempt to separate the political process from the management process in local government and in the NHS. But in practice, in both spheres, intention and reality can be, and especially in the NHS, are different. The managerial and the political domain become indistinguishable; politicians are drawn into the management domain and managers into the political.

The comparison between the NHS and local government remind us that the public sector should not be treated as a homogeneous entity. In the NHS, it is argued that there is a relatively clear separation of management and professional tasks, and a growing coalition between managers and politicians. This, it is argued, has meant a decline in professional power in terms of policy making, and processes of defining needs and resource allocation, but not in terms of control over people and areas of work. The evidence presented for this is not wholly convincing and is countered by that presented here in earlier chapters about the way in which the medical profession has adapted to the changed circumstances, so as to still exercise considerable power over key decisions. They argue that professional bodies in local government have successfully colonised managerial tasks and approaches.

Harrison and Nutley qualify their analysis of the situation in the NHS by stating that the established medical profession has lost least, nurses most. As in local government, front-line professionals have felt the most challenged, scrutinised, oppressed and marginalised. These areas of doubt and contradiction point up the need for continued research into these important questions.

The rationality and calculation associated with the new managerialism in the health service leads us to the concerns of our final concluding chapter on the future of the NHS. If all the attempts to reform the NHS are based on attempts to introduce rationality and efficiency in an attempt to achieve good health for all, to fulfil the modernist project, then what are the prospects for this in the future? Each reform was based on the modernist belief that there was an answer to the problems confronting the NHS. The evidence presented in this book suggests that there might not be.

In addressing this question we return to concept of 'citizenship' and 'the public good' and suggest that these might play a greater part in the way that health care is organised and delivered in the future. In this the relationship between professionalism and managerialism may be played out in a different context. It is an understanding of this relationship in the light of the wider debate that is addressed in the concluding chapter.

References

Bacharach, S. and Lawler, E. J. (1980), *Power and Politics in Organizations*, Josey-Bass, San Francisco.

Cox, D. (1991), 'Health Service Management - a sociological view: Griffiths and the non-negotiated order of the hospital', in Gabe, J. et al. (eds), *The Sociology of the Health Service*, Routledge, London.

Crook, S., Pakulski, J. and Waters, M. (1992), *Postmodernization. Change in advanced society*, Sage, London.

Department of Health and Social Security (1983), *The NHS Management Enquiry*, (Griffiths Report), HMSO, London.

Department of Health and Social Security (1987), *Promoting Better Health: The Governments Programme for Improving Primary Care*, HMSO, London.

Department of Health and Social Security (1989), *Working for Patients*, HMSO, London.

Fleck, L. (1979), 'Genesis and Development of a Scientific Fact' in Morton, R. K. (ed.), *Genesis and Development of a Scientific Fact*, University of Chicago Press.

Freidson, E. (1987), 'The Future of the Professions', *Journal of Dental Education*, 53: 140-144.

Glover, I. A. (1995), 'Professions at home and abroad: Now and in the future'. Paper presented to Cardiff Business School/ESRC Professionals in Late Modernity Seminar Series, No. 5, Imperial College.

Harrison, S., Hunter, D., Marnock, G. and Pollitt, C. (1992), *Just Managing: Power and Culture in the National Health Service*, Macmillan, Basingstoke.

Hunter, D. J. (1991), 'Managing Medicine: A Response to Crisis', *Social Science and Medicine*, Vol. 32, No. 4, pp. 444-49.

Keat, R. (1991), 'Consumer sovereignity and the integrity of practices', in Keat, R. and Abercrombie, N. (eds), *Enterprise Culture*, Routledge, London.

MacIntyre, A. (1990), *After Virtue: a study in moral theory*, Duckworth, London.

Morgan, G. (1990), *Organizations in Society*, Macmillan, London.

Sorge, A. (1978), 'The management tradition: a continental view', in, Fores, M. and Glover, I. A. *Manufacturing and Management*, HMSO, London.

Stewart, J. and Walsh, K. (1992), 'Change in the management of public services', *Public Administration*, 70, pp. 499-518.

2 In search of health and efficiency: the NHS 1948-1994

Michael Kelly and Ian Glover

Introduction

This chapter considers the organization and reorganizations of the British National Health Service (NHS) since its foundation. It is argued that not-with-standing claims to the contrary, there is a single line of evolution in the development of the provision of health care in Britain from the 1940s to the present. That line is based on three principles. First, that health services can be managed in a rational way. Second, that health care can be delivered efficiently. Third, that efficiency will produce health for the population at large. It is noted that the pace of change along that single line of development has quickened in recent years. However, speed should not be confused with direction. We argue for a single direction of development. We note that the rhetorics used with each successive reorganization have emphasised their differences from earlier systems of organization. Those rhetorics we suggest, have been designed to conceal rather than to illuminate. Finally, we suggest that the kind of efficiency which has been sought after, is Anglo-Saxon in origin and reflects the nature of development in British management thought over the last century or so.

The foundations of the National Health Service

It is possible to argue that the most recent changes in the NHS in Britain mark a fundamental shift from an administrative form of organization to a market-oriented one. We dispute this view, self-evident as it may appear to be and popular as it is with both the reformers and their political opponents. We argue instead, that the processes at work have a degree of continuity from events which may be traced back to the origins of the NHS. These were located in planning undertaken before the outbreak of the Second World War.

In the face of the threat of total war in the late 1930s, it was apparent to senior civil servants that there was a need for national organization and preparation. That planning had to extend to hospitals and health care. The ramshackle system, or non-system, of local authority hospitals, teaching hospitals, public health provision, voluntary hospitals and the rest, simply could not deal, it was believed, with the expected civilian and military casualties (Webster, 1988). As a result, a certain amount of systematic organization of hospital provision had begun some considerable time before planning for post-war reconstruction was contemplated.

When William Beveridge and his committee were appointed in 1941, they were able to draw upon the experience of this national planning. The attack on disease, heralded in Beveridge's report, was spearheaded by the national hospital system established before the war. In turn, this was based on the structures which had existed in the inter-war period, but tidied up and made more coherent and more rational and bureaucratic as a consequence of the needs of war-time. The hospital service coped well during hostilities, although casualties - civilian and military - were not as great as had been anticipated. Not unnaturally therefore, after the war the structure was built upon rather than dismantled (Ross, 1952).

The contemporary accounts make it clear that the arrangements for health care established in the NHS, as far as the hospital service was concerned, were not a decisive break with the past (Ross, 1952). It was the old pre-war set-up within a partly, but only partly, unified and rational structure. Thus after the hospital consultants had won various concessions, the patients were generally attending the same hospitals, and being treated and cared for by many of the same doctors and nurses as before the foundation of the NHS. Even so, the users' experiences were vastly different in the very important respect that the service was free at the point of delivery to everyone.

However - and this is our critical argument - a fundamental change had occurred in the rhetoric about health care delivery. The NHS was established by the Acts of Parliament of 1946 in England and 1947 in Scotland. The objective was to provide a comprehensive health service designed to secure improvement in the physical and mental health of the people and the prevention, diagnosis and treatment of illness (Section 1 of both Acts). What is significant about the objective laid out in Section 1 of the Acts, is that it assumes, that a health service which was able to secure the physical and mental health of the population was actually possible and that health in some general sense was within people's grasp. The establishment of the NHS was, if not an important structural departure, a very significant rhetorical change. In the relatively headily optimistic atmosphere of post-war Britain, at least as far as health was concerned, many people were encouraged to believe in the doctrine of improvement in health (Barnett, 1986). Thereafter, as other changes have been introduced in the NHS they have also been guided by the same principle of social engineering, albeit different forms of social engineering, which would create health for the population. The means to achieve it may have been different, but an underlying principle it had become never-the-less.

The Acts of Parliament which established the NHS assumed a technical and bureaucratic means, and above all a scientific facility which could be harnessed to bring about improvement in health. In historical terms the assumption associated with the Acts of Parliament marks the acknowledgement of a sea change in respect of health. No politician, and certainly no medical practitioner of the nineteenth century, would have dared to presume that medicine could achieve anything other than the amelioration of pain and suffering and then only imperfectly. Its job was not social engineering. While certain visionaries like Virchow (Ackernacht, 1981) and Chadwick (Flinn, 1965), or theorists like Comte (Aron, 1965) may have believed that the mastery of nature, and of disease, was ultimately possible, the empirical facts of the matter had always demonstrated the opposite. All through the nineteenth and well into the twentieth century medicine *qua* medicine had relatively modest aims.

However, by the time the NHS was established in 1948, the possibility of being able to overcome the scourge of illness seemed to be within reach of the population at large. Some politicians even believed that the NHS would be so effective as to reduce absolutely the amount of illness and hence the costs of the NHS to the nation. Although this, nor anything like it has happened (Black et al., 1988) the important belief was established that through human action in the form of social engineering and using scientific knowledge, health could be produced and illness eliminated. Here in the 1946 and 1947 Acts of Parliament, the principles of dominating nature and conquering disease are enshrined. By happy coincidence, antibiotics, the Salk vaccine and a great many public health reforms either became available or had become effective at about the same time or soon afterwards. These gave apparent and popular substance to belief in the inevitable progress of medicine. These were not, however, products of the NHS.

When it was established, the NHS had both a centralized and a local bureaucratic structure to achieve its aims. It was centralized because of the overall control of the Ministry of Health, and it was local at the level of delivery of services. In England and Wales the 1940s arrangements, which lasted until 1974, divided the country into fourteen regions for the purpose of hospital and specialized services while centrally the Minister of Health was responsible to Parliament for the NHS's work. Several other government departments had responsibilities for health too, but they had nothing directly to do with the National Health Service. These included, for example, the Ministry of Education which had charge of the health of school children. In each of the regions there was a Regional Hospital Board which planned and administered hospital and specialist services. Teaching hospitals in England remained separate from these arrangements and they were run by boards of governors directly responsible to the Minister of Health. In Scotland, both teaching and non-teaching hospitals were administered jointly by five regional hospital boards. Meanwhile, throughout England and Scotland, local authorities retained control of environmental health, social and preventive medicine and child health, and General Practitioners (medical and dental) were separate from the hospital and local authority services (Donaldson and Donaldson, 1983). The service was not in any sense completely unitary, the extent of national coverage of the population as a whole was uneven and local planning was fragmented (Acheson and Hagard, 1984).

The administrative system set up for the NHS in the 1940s was thus a product of its history. As we have noted, in 1948 the NHS, its staff, and its methods were those of the system that preceded it, and they were dominated by a particular administrative ethos. Although the establishment of a National Health Service was a political departure surrounded by much controversy (and one which subsequently became ideologically coded as the socialization of British medicine) the planning which had occurred in the immediate pre-war period, and the wartime experience itself had already established a *de facto* national service. Its structure and its functioning, were based upon the professional power of medical practitioners, the moral authority of nursing and a system of management which was borrowed from Imperial administration, local charitable and corporation munificence, and Civil Service procedures. It was underpinned by the State which had grown used to total control of resources borne out of war-time exigencies. There was *nothing* intrinsically socialistic, still less democratic, in any of these arrangements. The organizational pattern was typical of post-war and post-Imperial Britain, not withstanding a powerful and widely believed rhetoric based on principles of humane caring. These arrangements lasted with only minor revision until the mid-1970s.

The 1974 reorganization

In 1972, under Mr Heath's Conservative Government, a Reorganisation White Paper was published followed by the NHS Reorganisation Act of 1973 which took effect from 1st April 1974 (Webster, 1988). The 1974 reorganization was an attempt, amongst other things, to resolve the problems of a divided service at local level and its principal thrust sought to bring disparate elements together in a single administrative framework. In England and Wales, the Regional Hospital Boards, the hospital management committees, the Boards of Governors of the teaching hospitals, the family practitioner services, the services administered by local authorities (ambulances, epidemiology, family planning, health centres, health visiting, home nursing, midwifery, maternal and child health and preventive medicine) along with the school health services were all brought together. Only personal social services and environmental health were excluded and remained with local authorities. This system was organized into three tiers - regional, area and district. This phase of development may be characterised as searching for efficiency through rational bureaucratic means.

The 1974 reorganization was consequently the zenith of bureaucratic and centralizing tendencies of health service organization in Britain. It marks the point when locally elected governments were completely deprived of a role in health services. Those organizations, which had in effect been the back-bone of the provision of hospital and preventive services for more than a century, were finally overwhelmed by forces concentrating power in the centre, delegated to unelected, undemocratic and highly bureaucratic regional, area and district health authorities. The three tiers bore no necessary organic link to real geographical communities nor with traditional boundaries for the delivery of health, social or local government services. The logic of the 1974 reorganization was rationality and bureaucracy pushed to their limits. All, or nearly all, was within the embrace of one national organization. By all accounts the 1974 reorganization was disastrous, and the new system never worked properly. No sooner was it in place than the bureaucracy was shown to be dysfunctional. The three tiers were seen to be at least one tier too many. The tiers actually made planning more difficult than it had been hitherto. There was an elaborate consultative machinery between the three tiers and this complex and differentiated system proved to be mechanistic and highly formal. It was over-burdened with consultative committees. It also produced a tendency for a growth in the number of people employed who were not involved directly in patient care. The result was a dismal period in the history of the administration of the NHS. The loss of a locatedness in the local community and the absence of any significant democratic accountability must also be reckoned to be major problems. Some limited tinkering with the system took place during the Labour administration from 1974-1979 the attempt to redistribute resources under the RAWP formula (the Resource Allocation Working Party) and the introduction of cash limits in 1976, for example. However, the system itself was fundamentally unchanged.

Scotland escaped the English fate of three tiers in its 1974 reorganization. Its Regional Hospital Boards were abolished and all health services became the responsibility of the Secretary of State for Scotland. The Scottish Health Service was divided into Health Boards which combined the features of the regional, area and district administration found in England. The Boards were directly responsible to the Scottish Home and Health Department. GP services were also financed and directly administered by the Boards. Therefore, although Scotland was subject to the same centralizing tendencies, because of its smaller population it was not subject to the same bureaucratic structure.

General management

The next phase in the reorganization of the NHS began in 1982. The government had become concerned because not only had the new system cost £9 million to implement, but also it had failed to provide England and Wales with an effective framework for the delivery of care. Several further reforms were therefore instigated, principally the abolition of the area tier, the simplification of the consultative machinery and the introduction of unit management (Levitt and Wall, 1992).

However, no sooner was this under way than the next phase in reorganization began with the introduction of the principle of general management as enshrined in the Griffiths report (Department of Health and Social Security, 1983). What is critical about general management, is that it marked a self-consciously new departure in rhetoric. General management offered new solutions to old problems. Arguably the actual effects of Griffiths and the trend towards general management were less than was originally anticipated (Leathard, 1990). However, the philosophy of Griffiths reflected a new and distinct rationality namely that of Fayol-influenced managerialism. From 1948 at least, the governing rationality had been bureaucratic and administrative and the changes of 1974 were attempts to make the bureaucracy function in a bureaucratically more efficient way. Then in the 1980s the precept of proactive general management displaced the passive bureaucratic administration with a new set of principles in which *financial* (rather than service) efficiency was elevated from being one consideration in decision making, to *the* major policy objective. The battery of central activities associated with Griffiths like cash limits, manpower planning and annual reviews also reinforced the trend towards further centralization (Leathard, 1990).

The implementation of the principles of general management in the NHS involved the creation of a Health Services Supervisory Board (HSSB) at the Department of Health and Social Security (DHSS) in England, which was to decide on overall objectives, budgets and strategy. The board was to consist of the Secretary of State, the Minister of State for the NHS, the Permanent Secretary, the Chief Medical Officer, the Chairman of the Management Board and 2/3 non-executive members. Also at the centre, and below the HSSB the NHS Management Board was created. This was accountable to the HSSB, and chaired by a non-NHS civil servant.

The NHS Board was to have overall responsibility for running the NHS. All regional and district Health Authorities were to appoint their own General Managers who were to take charge of services at Regional and District level. Units would also be headed by General Managers (Leathard, 1990). The introduction of General Managers was supposed to facilitate planning, action and control, and the measurement of effectiveness and efficiency, qualities which Griffiths found lacking within the NHS (Ham, 1991). Griffiths had identified a lack of unified planning, implementation and control of performance, a failure to monitor performance, absence of direction, and the existence of so-called consensus management as major problems. Consensus management meant management by agreement and when agreement could not be reached it was passed for resolution to the next highest level of authority. In practice however, this seldom worked in an entirely mechanistic fashion, although difficult decisions did tend to be watered down (Ham, 1991). Instead of this the new General Manager was to be responsible, and accountable for decisions. Although Griffiths had not been given a remit in Scotland, on 10th November 1983 the Secretary of State for Scotland announced that all districts (although not all Scottish Health Boards had them) would be scrapped leaving Health Boards with subordinate units only.

Numerous criticisms have been, and were, levelled at the Griffiths approach. Aside from the fact that many commentators felt that there had been insufficient time for consultation, the implementation of general management seemed to produce yet another move towards centralized control, because of the increased role of the Civil Service in the management of the service. That said, Griffiths has also been criticized because organizationally, if not philosophically, it actually failed in its own terms. There was not an infusion of people from commerce and industry as had been intended, to take up general management posts and the great majority of appointments were from within the NHS. It has been suggested that erstwhile hospital administrators subverted the spirit of Griffiths. Many of those who did come in from commerce and industry left quickly. It has also been suggested that because of the speed of implementation little of real substance changed especially at district level. Worries were also expressed at the time about the possible loss of clinical freedom (Leathard, 1990).

Consumerism

The Griffiths managerialist ethos reigned supreme for a relatively short period. Then another, although not unrelated, rationality was elevated to prominence in the form of consumerism. This was identified in the White Paper, *Promoting Better Health*, published in November 1987. It laid out a series of objectives linking financial efficiency to a strong consumerist rhetoric. Its objectives were to make services more responsive to the needs of the consumer, to raise standards of care, to promote health and prevent illness, to facilitate choice and quality in primary care and to set clearer priorities for the family practitioner services (Department of Health and Social Security, 1987). Health care was a commodity to be consumed. Consumers exercised choice. The market in which to exercise those choices followed naturally enough.

Driven by the epidemiological evidence concerning diseases in which human behaviour plays a significant role, *Promoting Better Health* targeted a series of preventable diseases or health-damaging behaviours or states such as obesity, alcohol and drug misuse, smoking, dental disease and coronary heart disease. It argued 'Much of this distress and suffering could be avoided if members of the public took greater responsibility for looking after their own health. The government fully acknowledges its responsibility for raising individuals' awareness of the ways in which they can continue to take steps to maintain good health' (Department of Health and Social Security, 1987). With such a philosophy, health or illness is no longer the result of luck, chance or misfortune, but is a private duty. The State's responsibility is tempered with a new emphasis on individual responsibility.

Several changes to the organization of the service were therefore proposed. These were that there would be agreed targets for achieving higher levels of immunization and screening; there would be more health promotion sessions done by General

Practitioners; there would be regular and frequent health checks for particular sections of the community (children and the elderly); there would be a wider range of services available at the GP surgery; and there would be a new contract not only for GPs but also for dentists, to encourage more prevention. Most of these changes became operational for doctors on 1st April 1990, and dentists on 1st October the same year.

The next major changes in the NHS occurred in 1989 following the publication of *Working for Patients* (Department of Health, 1989). There are two major elements in *Working for Patients*. The first relates to financial arrangements and the second to re-emphasizing consumerism. *Working for Patients* may therefore be seen as a continuation of the rationalities of general management and consumerism, with the important additional proviso that the elements of the internal market would provide a counter-weight to the centralizing principles of the earlier policies.

The general aims of *Working for Patients* were to give better health care and more choice, and to increase satisfaction and rewards for those employed by the NHS. The objective was to cut waiting lists, make the appointments system work well, provide patients with information and introduce a new complaints procedure.

The main proposals for change were:

1   to delegate power and authority (including financial) to local levels in order to make the service more responsive to patients;

2   to set up self-governing hospital trusts which although within the overall structure of the NHS would earn revenue from the services they provided;

3   to allow money for patient treatment to cross administrative boundaries;

4   to create 100 new consultant posts;

5   to allow General Practitioners with more than 11,000 patients to apply for and run their own budgets; and

6   to set up vigorous auditing procedures to assess quality of service and value for money.

In order to put these proposals into practice another management structure was required. It was therefore to be the task of government to set a national framework of objectives and priorities. It would be the task of local management to get on with managing while remaining accountable. A new NHS Policy Board was created, chaired and appointed by the Secretary of State, to determine strategy, objectives and finances and to set objectives for a new body called the NHS Management Executive (NHSME). The NHS Policy Board was to replace the

HSSB. The NHSME was to be appointed by the Secretary of State to deal with operational matters within the national strategy. Regional Health Authorities (RHAs) were to ensure that government policy was carried out in their regions. The RHAs were to concentrate on setting performance criteria, monitoring performance and evaluating effectiveness. The Family Practitioner services were to be bought under the NHS Management Executive.

Before *Working for Patients*, the funding to District Health Authorities was based on a catchment allocation, with funding provided for their own hospitals. After *Working for Patients*, the funding was based on resident numbers, with care purchased for the population based on a weighted capitation formula. The allocation process flows from government to NHS, to Regional Health authorities to District Health Authorities and GP Fundholders and then on to hospital and community services.

The changes in funding under these arrangements were based on the operation of an internal market, divided into purchasers and providers. These 'purchasers' purchase care on behalf of the population from hospitals and other providers. At the centre of the market is the contracting process. Providers have to contract with various purchasers for the services they provide and then deliver those to budget. A hospital for example would have contracts with local and proximal Health Authorities, and GP Fundholders for different types of work. The types of work might include general surgery, urology, adult medicine and so on. Not all providers would provide everything. For the provider there would be targets for the different types of work and a critical task for the boards of directors of the new providers is to hit the target. If the targets are missed the budget may move into deficit.

The new NHS Trusts were defined as self-governing units within the NHS, with their own boards of directors. They have the freedom to organise their affairs within the overall statutory provisions. The main financial duties are to break even, to earn a return of 6 per cent on their capital, and to keep within their external financing limit. The Trust's performance is monitored by the NHS Management Executive whose outposts were to ensure that the Trusts met financial targets.

There were clearly defined relationships with the NHSME for the Trusts under the new system. However, the precise details of local financial systems were to be decided by the boards of the Trust. The boards would take financial advice from their directors of finance and chief executives. But within the broad parameters of public finance probity the boards were free to set up any systems they chose. Within this system the way in which contracts were devised and established was a matter for local discretion. The accounts of the Trusts have to be submitted to the Secretary of State, and the NHSME for external audit. Internally the finance director is obliged to report to the board on a bi-annual basis and at other intervals in respect of the financial health of the organization. The organization also had the power to establish various internal auditing arrangements in which the non-executive directors of the trust may have an important role.

During 1994 further developments occurred involving moves to more decentralization. The critical changes were: to create a clear identity for the NHS Management Executive within the Department of Health as the HQ of the NHS; to abolish the 14 statutory RHAs; reorganizing the NHSME to include 8 regional offices, each headed by a regional Director to replace both RHAs and the existing NHSME Outposts; to appoint non-executive members of the NHS policy board to cover each of the 6 regions; and to encourage DHAs and FHSAs to merge.

Thus within a relatively short space of time a range of new procedures, structures and organizations came into existence. New types of local and central managements have been formed, the methods of accounting and costing have been transformed, new systems developed and a great many administrative and managerial staff have moved or found the content of their work to be different. Consultants now practice working in an environment in which costs and contracts predominate. However, we argue that most if not all of this is surface change. In hospitals and in general practice, nurses and doctors minister to patients mostly in the same buildings, in much the same clinical way they have always done. The changes, like all the others, were driven by a search for the holy grail of efficiency. Management has become more frenetic and intense, but in reality much is as it always was.

British management thought and the NHS

The kinds of thinking which permeated the establishment of the NHS were firmly grounded in a British administrative tradition which developed in the nineteenth century. This was based on the notion that administration, and later, management, as a set of tasks and roles, should be set above other more specialist ones. This in turn had it roots in elite British preferences for government, intellectual activities, services and overseas trade over indigenous manufacturing and commerce (Barnett, 1972, 1986; Hampden-Turner, 1983; Glover, 1978; Middlemass, 1986; Sorge, 1979). The British commercial and imperial achievements which culminated in mid-Victorian economic supremacy and the acquisition of the world's largest and most far-flung empire by the 1920s, did not originally depend on the large-scale provision of technical and business expertise but upon these elite preferences and generalist notions.

Within the British Isles, management and organization had two main strands in the century or so which had the year 1900 as its mid-point, the metropolitan - administrative and the provincial-professional (Glover and Kelly, 1987, Chapter 9). They were opposed in key respects, but overlapped in others. The former had roots in public school and Oxbridge education, the Administrative Class of the Civil Service, the colonial service, medicine, law, the church and the military. It influenced large companies whenever public school and Oxbridge or similarly-educated generalists dominated their management, with professionals such as accountants and engineers supporting them from below with their specialist expertise. The latter tended to have less socially favoured roots, and very often partly in reaction against the previous one, it has been powerful in local government, in construction and in many medium-sized companies elsewhere and in the majority of nationalised industries and public utilities like the NHS.

The NHS was organised and managed from 1948 until 1974 very much along administrative-professional lines as we have shown. Its key professionals - the doctors - were, of course, very much cast in a sector specific mould. Its fragmented organization made it a somewhat unlikely candidate for proactive 'management', as distinct from more reactive administration. Its public service ethos, the prestige of doctors and nurses and of their tasks and its involvement, at the centre and/or top, with senior civil servants and politicians all contributed to helping the administrative-professional ideal to hold sway in the NHS long after it became unfashionable elsewhere. According to Barnett (1986) the creation of the NHS by using and adding to the piecemeal, inadequate and inequitably-distributed facilities in existence to the mid-1940s expressed much of the desire to build a postwar 'New Jerusalem' of full employment and cradle-to-grave social welfare which Britain could not afford but its idealistic politicians and civil servants were determined it should have.

The resistance of the NHS's 'professional monopolists' to 'corporate rationalisers' (Alford, 1975) has not just been a product of the power and prestige of scientific medicine. It has been underpinned by deeply-rooted cultural preferences for individual self-determination and for what Burrage (1973) called 'normative', as opposed to 'imperative' forms of occupation-formation and management, organization and control. These concern the influence of the notions of professionalism current when the NHS was founded. In many ways historical and other respects such notions are distinctly English, more than British, and more than simply Anglo-American (cf. Freidson, 1983). Burrage's discussion of the post-war Labour government's measures, which of course included the foundation of the NHS, offers some penetrating insights into the social and political character of British management. For him, there was a strong and very revealing intuitive element in the establishment of Britain's public corporations, nationalized industries and the NHS. Thus for many influential socialists including Tawney (1948) professional habits of self-discipline and peer judgements concerning quality of work offered a model of what relationships and behaviour should be like, one normally superior to the selfish individualism and pecuniary motivations inherent in the private sector. For Tawney, each public enterprise would be organized as a hierarchical amalgam of 'little societies; with each professional group given its assigned tasks and with all of them in their proper stations' (Tawney, 1948, p. 133). Internal and largely informal self-regulation of each group - with each enjoying a monopoly over its tasks and considerable autonomy - would minimise the need for external surveillance.

Such conservative ideals, for an organic society of hierarchically - ordered, self-governing collectivities and functional/occupational organization in industry, had much in common with Tawney's and other socialists' aims, even if Conservatives were less enthusiastic because of possible threats to individual liberty and responsibility. Burrage attributed this affinity between Conservative/conservative and socialist ideals to an underlying, 'enduring and widespread cultural preference' (Burrage, 1973, p. 256). He went on to note the predominantly monopolistic character of British public enterprise and corporations, which unlike France, Sweden, Italy and Canada, where only sections of industries or utilities had been brought under public ownership, complete or almost complete employment sectors or activities were nationalised. Burrage even went so far as to differentiate both professions and what he called classical public corporations from capitalist organizations insofar as only the first two were 'legal/customary monopolies, with fixed boundaries, based on a particular occupational activity'. He characterized public enterprise - and professions - in Britain by their 'fixed identity, [and] a certain moral unity resistant to technical or economic rationality by their autonomy from both executive and legislative power' (p. 259), and their lack of genuine accountability to consumers. Much of this had a significantly ad hoc, informal, ill-defined quality' and it all seemed more or less peculiar to Britain among the advanced industrial countries. Like professions, the public corporations were 'trusted' to provide the relevant services, although the latter were naturally compelled to adopt '*some* (our emphasis) bureaucratic characteristics to a limited degree.'

A major, widely-documented problem of mixed or matrix organization structures like that of the NHS is that the normally highly sensible management principle of unity of command is partly or completely abandoned in the pursuit of flexible and economic use of diverse abilities. Conflict, especially between functional/occupational and output/product criteria, tends to be endemic, and attempts to contain it can mean the bureaucracy which the adoption of a matrix structure was meant to dispense with reappears with a vengeance. This point is pertinent for understanding the history of the NHS; what began as a relatively autonomous and independent profession-dominated monopoly has evolved into a much more complex animal vulnerable to external pressures and bureaucratic interference from both outside and within its own ranks. Whereas its management in the 1950s had an administrative, sub-imperial tone, which emphasized consolidation and 'getting on with the job' (Klein, 1983) the following decades saw it increasingly influenced by growing proactive managerialist concern. Such concern was initially paternalistic, then technocratic, and then in the 1970s and after it became ideological and politicised, so that what was first conceived and administered as a tool of the state became a testing ground for different philosophies and accountability and management.

Although English individualism (cf. MacFarlane, 1978) seems to be at the root of a strong British preference for personal, occupational, established or enterprise-based solutions for organizational and managerial problems, corporatist tendencies on the part of the state have grown in time of perceived national emergency, as in the two World Wars and after the 1973 oil shock. Yet the resultant changes themselves tended, until 1979 at least, to embody faith in liberal compromise and to the loose-knit, paternalistic and reactive (cf. Barnett, 1972; Middlemas, 1979, 1986). Extremes of individualism and competition were mistrusted and in large public sector organizations there has been a tradition of managerial resistance to external supervision and inspection (Hanson, 1961). There have also been unresolved problems between professionals and administrators with professional departments becoming 'self-containing islands' (Shanks, 1963). It should however be remembered that bureaucratic control and work organization is by no means incompatible with the aspirations of professionals. It can give them both responsible autonomy (Freidman, 1977) and resources, even to the extent that professional 'best practice' and output and cultural control start to subvert bureaucratic authority (Child et al., 1983; Child, 1984). For most of the first decade of the existence of the NHS, Britain remained an imperial power, and until well into the 1970s British higher education was producing potential administrators and both traditional kinds of professional rather than business graduates or high-powered technocratic industrialists. Until the 1970s, managerialism was arguably quite a delicate child in Britain.

Even so, the NHS began to be more proactively managed in the 1970s than hitherto. However this did not mean that medical dominance of NHS management was inexorably worn away by corporate rationalism. Even in the 1990s doctors remain by far the single most powerful occupational group within the NHS. Consultants in hospitals and general practitioners in the community retain considerable clinical freedom and, within limits, managerial power.

Administrative consolidation and, in party-political terms, depoliticization, were the main experiences of the NHS until the 1960s from a management point of view. It was felt that so large an organization, and experiment, deserved and needed time to settle down, and administrative consolidation was simply, if increasingly, concerned with keeping costs down. Medical dominance was largely unchallenged and little was done to bridge the division between the hospital service on one hand and primary (GP) care and local authority services on the other, and the NHS was 'largely a hospital service' (Klein, 1983).

Klein went on to call the 1960s and the 1970s until the significant 1974 reorganization, an era of technocratic change for the NHS, with technocracy being the touchstone of modernization. There was a mix of innovation, expansion and rationalization, which included competition between the Conservative and Labour Parties about hospital building. The NHS was a full-blown technocracy in the sense of it being completely ruled as well as run by technical experts, but it was insofar as political debates about the NHS were more concerned with means than ends, with an ideology of efficiency and faith in organizational fixes for economic and political problems underpinning the positions of both major parties. More technically sophisticated forms of care such as renal dialysis and demographic changes such as growth in the numbers of the elderly meant that both the cost of the NHS and the demand for its services were growing faster than both spending and provision. Politicians and civil servants found powerful allies in clinical

27

autonomy and judgement when they wanted to ration expensive new techniques. Planning was continually developed, especially in the financial side, helping to engender a feeling that the centre had too little power in the NHS compared with its periphery. This atmosphere helped to produce the 1974 reorganization.

In any given employment sector most managers are specialists (in one sense almost all are, since the very idea of a sector means specialization) and most have had some kind of functional, occupational or professional specialist education and training and experience. These points highlight the fragility, in empirical terms, of the notion 'managerial'. Even the NHS general managers appointed following the Griffiths Report's implementation in 1984 whose backgrounds prior to entry were in (say) retailing or the armed forces were specialists in (the management of) health care, and the jobs of almost all doctors including GPs and especially of course consultants contain very important managerial elements.

The use of non-vocational university graduates and other non-health care specialists in NHS administration/management, and since the Griffiths Report, as specially-designated General Managers in a strengthened generalist planning-administration-control role, partly reflects traditional practices across a wide range of employment sectors in Britain with their preferences for 'amateur' generalists rather than the continental European-style technocrats such as by broadly educated and competent engineers in staffing senior posts. In this respect the NHS followed rather than led other major British employers like the Civil Service and larger private sector companies. In the context of Anglo-American thinking, professional monopolies, and corporate, even professional, management are often regarded as opposed phenomena, even if the terms 'professional management' and 'general management' are sometimes used interchangeably.

In a broader more culture-free sense, both English-language professionalism and managerialism may usefully and in part be understood as interdependent components of reactions, in certain English-speaking societies, to perceived difficulties in relationships between the world of higher education and work in manufacturing and commerce. In other words, each has had a flavour of closing the stable door after the horse of broadly educated high-powered technocrats had bolted. Because education had not delivered such people, industry and commerce had to make do with ex-Oxbridge and similar non-vocational graduate generalists and not always sector-oriented professionals or specialist accountants, engineers and so on. As a sort of temporary remedy, perhaps both types have been offered generalist management training to make generalist managers more professional and narrow professionals more broadly based and better equipped. Unlike most of British industry and commerce, health care in Britain has always been almost entirely professional-dominated, with the dominant professional grouping always a very high-status one. Unlike salaried engineers and accountants in industry and commerce, the work and employment situations of doctors approximate far more closely to those of the traditional independent fee-taking service-to-individual-client ideal, providing the service free and with a sense of responsibility to the local community (cf. Glover, 1978). However the size, unwieldiness, cost, complexity and dependence on the state of the NHS have made it especially vulnerable to changes in managerial and political fashions. Numerous fashions or models of management have influenced British management since 1945, and the NHS too, but the most important distinction between the approaches for us to note at present is that between hard and soft versions of Anglo-Saxon arm's length managerialism (cf. Pahl and Winkler, 1974; Glover and Martin, 1986). The former is predominantly financial and rationalistic in its concerns, the latter being imbued with Mayoite paternalism. The management of the NHS has generally moved from soft to hard in such terms, although the reasons for, rationales, content and effects of the relevant changes in organizing structures, staff, funding, resource allocation and so on have been very diverse and complicated.

The persistence of the administrative-professional approach in the NHS was, and is, due to a mixture of three major influences. There has been the sheer size and complexity, and the fragmented and unco-ordinated character of the organization itself, making radical change hard to implement, and combining with the generalist, partly amateur nature of top management, which involves politicians, civil servants and outsiders, to make the whole ethos and approach of top management tend towards the passive. Medical dominance and medical prestige have persisted partly because of the extremely high levels of the skill and knowledge of doctors, and partly because doctors are so obviously and simply so important to health care, irrespective of any criticisms that can be made about their relationships with other health professionals, patients and the wider society. Finally the NHS has remained a highly popular organization as far as the general British public is concerned both for what it does and as a source of national pride and this very general fact is itself a source of inertia.

In some ways, although only some, the NHS has been an organization run on Continental-style technocratic lines. Most of its management has been dominated by technical experts, meaning doctors and nurses and other professional specialists. Doctors, the dominant group of specialists, are rather like senior engineers in continental countries like France and Germany insofar as their lengthy education and training, pre-clinical and clinical, is similar. However, the organization of education has almost always been significantly narrower than that of Continental engineers and they have, in general, been educated, trained, and employed as prestigious super-technicians of a kind, not as technocrats who are capable of handling *all* aspects of the financial, human resource and commercial as well as technical management of their sector.

Conclusion

The evolution of the NHS, we suggest, has been driven by the twin concerns of modernism -the liberation of humanity and the conjunction of the scientific and the political towards the solution of the efficiency problem (Lyotard, 1984). The organizational principles underlying the structure of the NHS may have been originally administrative, become increasingly bureaucratic and eventually apparently market-driven, but it is nonetheless the case that at each successive reorganization the modernist belief that an answer existed to organizational problems, was paramount.

It is often argued that the changes which the NHS is currently undergoing are fundamental and radical, and amount to a transformation of a bureaucratically administered service to a market and consumer driven business. This chapter has taken a contrariwise position. It is argued that the most recent reorganization is little more than the extension of an organizational principle which has been at work since the foundation of the NHS. This is that it is possible to manage the delivery of health care services efficiently through some kind of organizational framework. It is further suggested that the rhetorics which have surrounded the various organizations and reorganizations have themselves been deceptive. The traditions dominating British management, and which have been invoked at each reorganization, are also historically rooted. Each new reform has claimed to have the answer to the question of the provision of health via the delivery of health care. This, we suggest is rhetorical and ideological, because it purports to show that the latest version or reorganization is both different and better than its predecessor. We argue that this disguises the much more important similarities between all the reorganizations, including the most recent. These similarities that are a belief that answers to organizational problems exist - or at least can be found if enough technical or other expertise is pushed at the problem, and that advanced societies (including their health care delivery systems) are on an onward and upward path of improvement which is more or less infinite, and that administrative structures of one kind or another can achieve ultimate perfection - in this case a healthy population.

This we suggest is a fallacy. It is fallacy because health for all, or a healthy nation, are simply unattainable given present medical knowledge and stubborn inequalities in health (Black et al., 1988; Whitehead, 1988). It is also a fallacy because it is based on a rationalist assumption that through social engineering or market forces health can be achieved (Kelly and Charlton, 1995). The reality, has been a series of changes in the organization which have had singularly little difference to the health of the nation. The major improvements in the health of the nation which have occurred, have done so because of better housing, improved nutrition, greater immunisation coverage, better medical technology, more efficacious drugs, more health education, and the reduction in levels of smoking in the population, none of which have anything to do with the managerial ethos or structure of the NHS.

The most serious fallacy which has dominated the various reorganizations, is the fallacy that a large and complex system such as the NHS, is ultimately efficiently manageable. Managerialists, reformers and proponents of internal markets, may each have something interesting to say, but translated into the day to day reality of managing the unmanageable they are forever destined to fail. That is not of course to say that systems of controls, budgeting, strategic vision and human resource management are not required. Quite the contrary. Organizations have to be managed. Our argument is with the notion that in a service so large and so complex and diverse as the NHS, containing conflicting professional groups, a wide variety of functions and dealing with the general public as its client group, there is an ultimate answer to the efficiency problem. The best that can probably be attained is to strive to minimise inefficiency. Unfortunately each of the reorganizations we have described claimed to have the answer and that their answer would make a difference to people's health. Consequently a kind of hyperactive culture of change now infuses the Health Service in search of things which are quite unobtainable in any meaningful sense. There are physical, personal, technical and resource limitations as to what can be achieved with health care. Containment of contingencies in a way in which people may be rendered *healthier* but not healthy in an absolute sense, is probably the best that can be hoped for. The reams of paper and the millions of pounds that have been expended in trying to prove otherwise beggar belief.

More limited objectives than ultimate health for all might have helped patients rather more than the hyperactivity of recent years. In the end what we seem to have been left with is change for change's sake. It is almost as if the ultimate telos has been lost and activity towards continual change has become a goal in itself. We do have a range of narratives to call upon to justify the changes from Beveridge's original founding principles, to the operation of the internal market. We suggest that all these reforms are forms of narrative. Given the impossibility of the task to hand, that is all they ever could be (Vattimo, 1988).

References

Acheson, R.M. and Hagard, S. (1984), *Health Society and Medicine: An Introduction to Community Medicine*, Blackwell, Oxford.

Ackernacht, E. (1981), *Rudolf Virchow*, Arno Press, New York.

Alford, R. (1975), *Health Care Politics*, University of Chicago Press, London.

Aron, R. (1965), *Main Currents in Sociological Thought*, (trans.), Howard, R. and Weaver, H. Penguin, London.

Barnett, C. (1972), *The Collapse of British Power*, Eyre Methuen, London.

Barnett, C. (1986), *The Audit of War*, Macmillan, London.

Black, D., Morris, J., Smith, C. and Townsend, P. (1988), 'The Black Report', in *Inequalities in Health*, Penguin, London.

Burrage, M. (1973), 'Nationalisation and the Professional Ideal', *Sociology*, Vol 7, pp. 252-72.

Child, J. (1984), *Organization: A Guide to Problems and Practice*, 2nd edition, Harper and Row, New York.

Child, J., Fores, M., Glover, I. and Lawrence, P. (1983), 'A Price to Pay? Professionalism and Work Organization in Britain and West Germany', *Sociology*, Vol. 20, pp. 63-78.

Department of Health and Social Security (1983), *The NHS Management Enquiry* (Griffiths Report), HMSO, London.

Department of Health and Social Security (1987), *Promoting Better Health: The Government's Programme for Improving Primary Care*, HMSO, London.

Department of Health (1989), *Working for Patients*, HMSO, London.

Donaldson, R. and Donaldson, L. (1983), *Essential Community Medicine*, MTP, Lancaster.

Flinn, M.W. (ed.), (1965), *Report on the Sanitary Condition of the Labouring Population of Great Britain, by Edwin Chadwick, 1842*, Edinburgh University Press, Edinburgh.

Friedman, A.L. (1977), *Industry and Labour: Class Struggle at Work and Monopoly Capitalism*, Macmillan, London.

Freidson, E. (1983), 'The Theory of Professions', in Dingwall, R. and Lewis, P. (eds.), The *Sociology of the Professions*, St Martins, London.

Glover, I.A. (1978), 'Professionalism and Manufacturing Industry', in, Fores, M. and Glover, I.A. *Manufacturing and Management*, HMSO, London.

Glover, I.A. and Kelly, M.P. (1987), *Engineers in Britain:A Sociological Study of the Engineering Dimension,* Allen and Unwin, London.

Glover, I.A. and Martin, G. (1986), 'Managerial Work An Empirical and Cultural Contradiction in Terms?', Paper presented at the 1986 British Sociological Association Conference, Loughborough.

Ham, C. (1991), *The New National Health Service: Organization and Management*, Radcliffe, Oxford.

Hampden-Turner, C. (1983), *Gentlemen and Tradesmen: The Values of Economic Catastrophe*, Routledge and Kegan Paul, London.

Hanson, A.M. (1961), *Parliament and the Public Ownership*, Cassell, London.

Harrison, S. and Pollitt, C. (1994), *Controlling Health Professionals the Future of Work and Organization in the NHS,* Open University Press, Buckingham.

Kelly, M.P. and Charlton, B.G. (1995), 'The Modern and the Post Modern in Health Promotion', in, Bunton, R., Nettleton, S. and Burrows, R. (eds.), *The Sociology of Health Promotion and the New Public Health*, Routledge, London.

Klein, R . (1983), *The Politics of the National Health Service,* Longman, London.

Leathard, A. (1990), *Health Care Provision: Past, Present and Future*, Chapman and Hall, London.

Levitt, R. and Wall, A. (1992), *The Reorganized National Health Service*, 4th edition, Chapman and Hall, London.

Lyotard, J-F. (1984), *The Post-Modern Condition A Report on Knowledge*, (trans.), Bennington, G. and Massum, B. Manchester University Press, Manchester.

Macfarlane, A. (1978), *The Origins of English Individualism: The Family Property and Social Transition*, Blackwell, Oxford.

Middlemas, K. (1979), *Politics in Industrial Society,* Andre Deutsch, London.

Middlemas, K. (1986), *Power, Competition and the State: Vol. 1, Britain in Search of Balance*, Macmillan, Basingstoke.

Pahl, R. and Winkler, J. (1974), 'The Economic Elite: Theory and Practice', in Stanworth, P. and Giddens, A. *Elites and Power in British Society*, Cambridge University Press, Cambridge.

Ross, J.R. (1952), *The National Health Service in Great Britain: An Historical and Descriptive Study*, Oxford University Press, Oxford.

Shanks, M. (1963), (ed.), *The Lessons of Public Enterprise*, Cape, London.

Sorge, A. (1979), 'Engineers in Management: A Study of the British, German and French Traditions', *Journal of General Management*, Vol. 5, pp. 45-57.

Tawney, R.M. (1948), *The Acquisitive Society*, Harcourt, New York.

Vattimo, G. (1988), *The End of Modernity: Nihilism and Hermeneutics in Post-Modern Culture*, (trans.), Snyder, J.R., Polity, Cambridge.

Webster, C. (1988), *The Health Services Since the War: Volume 1 Problems of Healthcare: The National Health Service Before 1957*, HMSO, London.

Whitehead, M. (1988), 'The Health Divide', in, *Inequalities in Health*, Penguin, London.

Part II

COMMODIFICATION

3 Human resource managers as professionals in managing change in NHS trusts

Colin Bryson, Michael Jackson and John Leopold

Introduction

This chapter examines the role of personnel and human resource managers in the NHS, especially in NHS Trusts. The role of human resource managers in the managing people and employment relations aspects of the move to NHS Trust status is analysed against theories of personnel managers as initiators and influencers of change, and in the context of personnel staff in the NHS as professionals in an organization dominated by professionals.

We therefore examine the literature on strategies for human resource managers to engineer change, then review the key features of employment relations in the NHS before NHS Trusts, and draw upon our research into 19 NHS Trusts in Great Britain, and other recently published evidence to demonstrate the lack of progress compared with the expectations of government ministers and many of those involved in NHS management. Finally, we try to explain this lack of progress in terms of the models of personnel management advanced in the earlier section.

Strategies for human resource managers

Legge (1978) has identified two key strategies available for personnel managers as a way of increasing their influence within organisations; the conformist innovator and the deviant innovator. The conformist innovator identifies with the objective of organizational success, emphasizing cost benefit and conforming to the criteria adopted by managerial colleagues, who usually have greater power. The deviant innovator, on the other hand, identifies with a set of norms that are distinct from, but not necessarily in conflict with, the norms of organizational success. Power derives from an independent, professional stance for working with managerial clients (Torrington, 1991). In analysing the relationship between HRM and the personnel function, Torrington went on to argue that:

> conformist personnel management innovators do no more than reflect the competencies and values of their colleagues. Deviant personnel innovators are able to make a distinctive contribution to the totality of management, which becomes richer and more resourceful as a result. (p. 66).

Armstrong (1991) observes that 'conformist innovation' implies the adaptation of personnel practice to the requirements of control and reporting systems, (p. 158). It therefore requires the personnel department to supply hard data, to attempt to justify personnel activity itself in cost terms and, possible to develop human asset accounting as a means of solving both of the problems simultaneously. 'Deviant innovation' would by contrast challenge the accounting frame of reference itself.

An alternative, but related, typology is that of Tyson and Fell (1986) who offer a threefold hierarchical typology of personnel management:

1   The Clerk of Works: personnel management carried out as administrative support, reactive to the needs of other managers and carrying little authority.

2   The Contracts Manager: seeks to react to need by deploying procedures and systems rather than being only spontaneous.

3   The Architect: seeks to build the organisation as a whole and works within the dominant coalition of the organisation.

Having outlined these models, which may help us to understand the nature of human resource management in the NHS, we must now turn to review the evidence about the role of personnel management in the NHS, how this might have changed with the advent of NHS Trusts and the extent to which the models let us understand the pace and variation of change in key indicators in the Trusts.

One indication of the likely role of personnel management in NHS Trusts came from the then Personnel Director of the NHS Management Executive, Eric Caines, (Spry and Caines, 1991, p. 25):

> The extent to which senior personnel staff can get close to general managers and work with them will be the touchstone of whether the best possible and most effective policies can be developed. There will need to be mutual confidence between the two.

This seems to tie in with Legge's model of the conformist innovator. It suggests that NHS personnel managers can only succeed if they are linked closely with general managers and share the same values and policies. Indeed Caines went on to criticize existing personnel management in the NHS:

> Up to now, under the highly centralised systems operated by the Department of Health and by regional and district health authorities, personnel managers at unit level have had little to offer general managers, who in turn have came to regard their personnel departments as being concerned merely with the local administration of centrally prescribed arrangements and centrally determined agreements.

In short, Caines saw the majority of personnel staff fitting into Tyson and Fell's 'Clerk of Works' category, or at best the 'contracts manager'. Indeed Caines doubted if all existing personnel managers could develop into lead players doing 'a fully rounded professional job' in the new Trusts.

These themes have been taken up by Guest and Peccei (1992) in their study of NHS personnel staff. They differentiated between three levels of personnel work - personnel administration, professional personnel management and human resource management. Personnel administration is seen as being driven mainly by concerns for effective administration and cost minimisation, whereas HRM is seen as being concerned with making full use of human resources. They concluded that personnel management in the NHS is currently performing most effectively at level 1 (personnel administration) and has some considerable distance to travel before it can be described as effectively practising human resource management (p. 24). They further reveal that personnel departments have considerably less influence over major policy decisions than over either major personnel decisions or day to day personnel decisions (p. 26).

These findings echo the view of the Griffiths report (DHSS, 1983) a decade earlier which recommended the appointment of a Personnel Director to the new NHS Management Board, and implying some criticisms of existing health service personnel officers, recommended that the person be appointed initially from outside the NHS and the Civil Service (para 22). The agenda for the new Personnel Director included securing the full commitment and involvement of staff. Also high on the agenda was the devolution of personnel matters and a close working relationship between personnel and line management. Thus for Griffiths:

> The most important development to be achieved is one of morale and attitudes. This will be done by the line management leadership, and the perceived professional competence of the Personnel Director and an injection of enthusiasm and pride in the quality of service provided (para 24).

However, Guest and Peccei also discovered that:

> the units which tend to be most effective in terms of the management of human resources are ones in which there is a close partnership between personnel and other functions at the top of the organisation, leading to a high

degree of policy integration (p. 43).

This again ties in with Legge's 'conformist innovator' model. Significantly they did not find that personnel effectiveness was related to key characteristics of personnel such as the size, resourcing and professionalisation of the personnel department. Indeed they conclude:

> that improvements in personnel management effectiveness are likely to depend less on such things as the increased professionalisation and resourcing of personnel, than on the development of a closer partnership between personnel and line management (p. 46).

The suggestion is then, that the most effective strategy for human resource managers in the NHS is the 'conformist innovator' one. This implies that personnel/human resource management professionals should seek to ally themselves with both the goals of the organisation and with senior managers who are key in determining these and in securing their implementation. This corresponds with Tyson and Fell's architect model. We should expect to find such human resource managers seeking to justify their contribution in quantitative terms. By contrast, we should not expect to find many examples of 'deviant' innovation, based on an independent professional stance.

If NHS Trust human resource directors were to adopt a 'conformist innovator/architect model, then they would have to be clear about which was the dominant coalition in the organisastion to align themselves with. In NHS Trusts this is not necessarily obvious as there is a potential conflict between the managerialism of post Griffiths' general management, now manifest in the chief executives of Trusts, and the traditional professionalism of the NHS manifest through the key professional groups, but above all doctors.

On the other hand if the 'deviant innovator' approach were to be adopted it is perhaps unlikely that potential champions of such an approach would be found already working in NHS personnel management. We have cited various pieces of research and commentary which indicate the majority of NHS personnel managers are not in the architect mode. In order to implement the agenda associated with general management and the purchaser/provider split, it was perhaps necessary to bring in human resource specialist with experience of managing change in other organisations. Such experience combined with professional credentials should outweigh any lack of NHS specific experience.

The debate as to whether insiders or outsiders are more appropriate in the NHS has arisen in earlier NHS reorganisations and the evidence shows that it has been resolved decisively in favour of insiders - those who have spent their career in the NHS, even if they have not always been in personnel/human resources (Leopold & Beaumont, 1985). Analysing the backgrounds of NHS personnel officers in Scotland they concluded that:

The dominant type of personnel officer in the NHS is the 'late professional' who moved into a personnel post from the Service. Consistent with our earlier argument that 'insiders' are less likely to need to demonstrate 'professionalism' by acquisition of professional institute membership, only about a third of personnel officers are IPM members (p. 224).

Since the 1983 reorganisation, and more particularly post *Working for Patients* and the creation of the internal market there has been a tendency to recruit managers from outside the NHS. In an article in the *Health Service Journal*, (10 June 1993) Davies suggested that 'the NHS's fixation with recruiting managers from outside its own ranks has burgeoned steadily since the mid 1980s.' He indicated that while some outsiders were making their mark in the NHS, that also 'it is equally certain significant numbers are experiencing the difficulties of acclimatization' (p. 24).

The human resource directors in our sample of Trusts were overwhelmingly from an NHS background. Some had a mixture of NHS and private sector experience, but only a few were recruited directly from a private sector background. There is still strong support for the insider approach. One Trust Director of Personnel has highlighted the importance of NHS specific knowledge if personnel staff are to integrate their skills and knowledge with the concerns of general management, by combining process and business skills into an 'expert plus' role to make a real contribution to the whole planning process:

> The framework implies that a combination of certain key skills, professional expertise and service knowledge is required before an adviser with a personnel background can have the credibility to influence service planning decisions at the earliest stages' (Munro, 1992, p. 24).

According to Guest and Peccei (1992) only about a quarter of NHS personnel department staff have IPM qualifications. This is similar in Trusts and DMUs, although Trusts have a higher proportion currently studying for IPM qualifications. This evidence does not indicate a movement of professionally qualified staff into NHS personnel departments and suggests that the 'deviant innovator' strategy is not to be found in the Service.

Employment relations pre NHS trusts

We turn now to examine the key features of employment relations in the NHS prior to the advent of Trusts and then draw evidence from our survey of nineteen Trusts to assess the extent to which changes have been introduced and the role of human resource managers in this.

The Trusts (listed in Table 3.1) were chosen for research for a variety of reasons, but the principal one was that most of them were known to be, or at least claimed to be, at the forefront of change on attaining trust status. The trusts covered a geographical spread from the North of Scotland to the South-West of England. Size, by numbers employed, varied from over 7,000 to fewer than 300, and the range of services covered varied from ambulance trusts, through specialist mental health and mental handicap services, to large general hospitals. Documentary evidence was consulted and interviews were conducted by the research team with senior managers, usually Human Resources or Personnel Directors between May 1992 and June 1993. It is not suggested that the trusts looked at are a representative sample, but if new employment relationships were being adopted in NHS Trusts, then they should be found in this sample. Similarly if human resource directors were influencing change significantly, then these Trusts would be excellent examples of this.

A main feature of the pre-trust NHS was that pay and conditions of employment were determined nationally. This was either through Pay Review Bodies (doctors and dentists; nurses and midwives; professions allied to medicine (PAMs), through Whitley Councils (administrative and clerical staffs; ancillary staffs; ambulance staff and professional and technical 'B' staff), or direct negotiation with the Department of Health (maintenance staff). Even where pay was determined via Pay Review Bodies, in many cases Whitley councils also existed to determine conditions of employment. The negotiated agreements tended to be very prescriptive and applied uniformly throughout the country with no account taken of variations in labour markets (except for London allowances). Within health authorities and boards, the role of the personnel department was to interpret the detailed agreements and to ensure their application. The system had a number of critics and various attempts were made to refine or improve it. These included a review of the system by Lord McCarthy (1976), a later review by the TUC (1982) and an attempt to involve the managers and employers in the service more in pay determination through Whitley (Leopold and Beaumont, 1986). A major problem in the system was the relationship between the central government departments (Health and Social Security and the Scottish Office) and the employing authorities over control of staff costs which constitute over seventy per cent of NHS costs. This relationship was summed up by McCarthy as 'employers who do not pay and paymasters who do not employ' (McCarthy, 1976).

Throughout the 1980s, the Conservative Government sought to introduce the operation of market forces into various parts of the public sector. In terms of pay determination the government objected to it being determined nationally providing a uniform rate for a particular job which applied throughout the country, no matter the state of the local labour market. In their 1988 White Paper the government argued that pay structures would have to change:

Table 3.1
Case study NHS trusts
Staff complement and trust services

Trust	established	staff	service provision
Aberdeen	April 1st, 1992	5000	large general & small hospitals, multisite
Bradford	April 1st, 1991	4000	large general &small hospitals, multisite
CMH	April 1st, 1991	1526	general hospital on one site
CA	April 1st, 1992	300	ambulance service
Homewood	April 1st, 1991	975	mental health & handicap(small acute unit and community)
MCHCC	April 1st, 1991	7000	large general &small hospitals, multisite, community care
MH	April 1st, 1991	2400	general and small hospital, 2 sites, community care
Norfolk	April 1st, 1991	460	ambulance service
NAS	April 1st, 1991	750	ambulance service
Premier	April 1st, 1992	2400	mental health & handicap, small acute units, community care
RNOH	April 1st, 1991	650	specialist acute services, 2 sites
RSNH	April 1st, 1993	1100	specialist mental handicap, (hospital and community)
SAH	April 1st, 1992	1950	large general & small hospitals, 3 sites
Southend	April 1st, 1991	2700	large general hospital
SRI	April 1st, 1993	1700	general hospital and small hospital, 2 sites
ULTH	April 1st, 1991	5000+	large general & small hospitals, multisite
WDGH	April 1st, 1991	2200	general hospitals, 3 sites
WDMH	April 1st, 1991	700	mental health (community)
Weston	April 1st, 1991	1300	general hospital, mental health, community care

Aberdeen Royal Hospitals NHS Trust	Aberdeen
Bradford Hospitals NHS Trust	Bradford
Central Middlesex HospitaL NHS Trust	CMH
Cleveland Ambulance NHS Trust	CA
Homewood NHS Trust	Homewood
Manchester Central Hospitals and Community Care NHS Trust	MCHCC
Mid-Cheshire Hospitals NHS Trust	MH
Norfolk Ambulance NHS Trust	Norfolk
Northumbria Ambulance NHS Trust	NAS
Premier Health Trust	Premier
Royal National Orthopaedic Hospital NHS Trust	RNOH
Royal Scottish National Hospital NHS Trust	RSNH
South Ayrshire Hospitals NHS Trust	SAH
Southend Healthcare NHS Trust	Southend
Stirling Royal Infirmary NHS Trust	SRI
United Leeds Teaching Hospitals NHS Trust	ULTH
West Dorset General Hospitals NHS Trust	WDGH
West Dorset Mental Health NHS Trust	WDMH
Weston Area Health NHS Trust	Weston

There is no uniquely right way of determining pay but existing approaches to pay bargaining, beloved of trade unions and employer alike, will need to change if we are to achieve the flexibility essential to employment growth. (Department of Employment, Cmd. 540, 1988, p.23).

They then went on to point in more detail to the problems associated with the current methods of pay determination - "In particular the 'going rate', 'comparability' and 'cost of living increases' are outmoded concepts". It was argued that more attention had to be paid to individual performance and especially ability to pay. The decentralization of bargaining clearly was seen as a way of moving in the required direction.

The government therefore encouraged many initiatives throughout the public sector, and especially on privatisation, which would introduce local labour market variations into pay determination. One example of this in the NHS was when the new grade of Health Care Assistant was established in 1990, the NHS Management Executive decreed that their terms and conditions of employment would be determined locally and they would not be covered by any existing Whitley Council. Similarly general and senior managers do not have their pay determined through collective bargaining but set by the Department of Health and have a substantial measure of performance related pay built into it. However these development only nibble at the edges of pay determination for the vast majority of NHS staff. It is the creation of NHS Trusts which opens up the potential for significant change in both the locus and the content of pay determination in the NHS. This potential was welcomed by government and senior managers in the NHS.

Criticisms of national pay determination were made by virtually all of the human resource managers we interviewed in the course of our study. These included the belief that national arrangements do not take account of local conditions, perspectives or needs. There was a feeling, particularly from Trusts geographically distant from London, that national arrangements were driven by London concerns which were not relevant to the rest of the country. Other important criticisms were also made; the arrangements and outcomes are inflexible and complex; there is no link to individual or group performance or the ability to reward enhanced performance, competency or flexibility; local managers have little influence on the outcome and this is an abrogation and diminishing of their responsibility; there are a large number of separate negotiations based on occupational groups and this reinforces unfair differences in pay and conditions.

Given this catalogue of criticisms of the old system, it is no surprise to find that many human resource managers, trust chief executives and other executive directors were enthusiastic about the potential for change that trust status opened up. Before going on to examine this, we must first add a rider; this enthusiasm was not universal. Some managers saw virtue in the national arrangements - they saved costs by avoiding replication of pay determination machinery; they provided a protective net for low paid staff; helped to ensure equity and maintain stability; and that they insulated local managers from the blame for low pay awards.

On balance however, the managers we interviewed favoured the ending of national arrangements and welcomed the ability of Trusts to determine pay and conditions for trust staff locally. Local pay determination, it was believed, would enable Trusts to develop a local response to the labour market; to implement a reward strategy appropriate to, and devised by, Trusts; to reward performance or flexibility. Local determination is expected to enable the organisation to have greater flexibility in a broader sense, including the containment of costs. There is a cultural dimension with an emphasis on more identification with the trust an the staff more directly sharing in organisational goals and successes.

The potential for change under trust status is not confined to the determination of pay. Other terms and conditions of employment would no longer necessarily be as laid down by Whitley, but could be established locally. These could include grading systems, job evaluation, common pay spines, equal opportunities policies, changes in skill mix and the harmonisation of condition of employment across all employee groups. Trusts are not required to follow the structure of the various Whitley Councils in establishing consultation and bargaining arrangements. They are not even obliged to determine pay through collective bargaining; but if they chose that route are not required to recognise all 36 national organisations active in the Whitley Council system and have freedom to develop bargaining units appropriate to the overall strategy of the trust.

In the initial euphoria of impending trust status a variety of ideas were being canvassed as being appropriate for the new era. These included single pay spines for all staff from cleaners to consultants; cafeteria benefits so that different mixes could be agreed appropriate to be career and status position of the recipient; and abolition of incremental scales and their replacement by spot salaries with increases being tied to performance.

Table 3.2
Proportion of staff on trust determined conditions in case study trusts

Trust	approach to transfer	reward strategy introduction	% all staff on trust conditions 1991	1992	1993	AMJ
Aberdeen	not pushing	phased				70
Bradford	not pushing	not yet			15	
CMH	not pushing	phased			60	
CA	proactive	big bang	I50-60	35	77	
Homewood	proactive	big bang			52	65
MCHCC	not yet	phased				N/A
MH	targeting	phased			25	
Norfolk	active	mixture			30	I
NAS	proactive	big bang	I60	85		98

46

	Approach to transfer	Reward strategy introduction	% staff on trust contracts
Premier	not priority	phased	3
RNOH	collectively	mixture	100 I
RSNH	not pushing	phased	
SAH	targeting	phased	27 1 40
Southend	targeting	phased	5 18
SRI	not pushing	not yet	26 8
ULTH	not pushing	not yet	I
WDGH	active	phased	15 35
WDMH	not pushing	big bang	25 35
Weston	targeting	phased	13(+17)

Explanatory Notes

Approach to transfer - a measure of the degree to which trust managers are encouraging staff to sign local trust contracts

Reward strategy introduction - method of introducing local conditions of service

% staff on trust contracts - figure on given date, I implementation of new reward local package/structure

(Weston includes second % showing staff on trust contracts but still under Whitley pay determination)

Changes in human resource management practices in NHS trusts

After four years of experience of NHS Trusts, the initial euphoria about radical change in employment conditions has died down. A number of managers have become disillusioned about the extent and pace of change in the NHS, none more so than Eric Caines, then personnel director of the NHS Management Executive, whose reasons for resigning were widely publicised. Commenting on the failure of NHS Trusts to devise Trust-based reward systems balancing fair pay and the need for flexibility in work practices, he said:

> Unfortunately, and it grieves me to say this, the NHS has almost certainly passed up the best, indeed the only opportunity it has ever had to make fundamental changes in these areas.' (Financial Times 23.3.93).

Changes in pay determination

As has been indicated earlier, one of the key areas where the government hoped for change in NHS Trusts was in the area of pay determination. Trusts are not required to adopt Whitley or Pay Review Body terms and conditions for their staff, but are able to establish their own local forms of pay determination. The evidence from our research is that, with some exceptions, progress towards the widespread adoption of locally determined pay and condition of service has been slow. The detail of this is shown in Table 3.2. Two points stand out from this table. Firstly, that very few Trusts have achieved anything like the majority of their staff on Trust terms and conditions. This finding supports that of an IRS (1993) survey which found that the proportion of staff in each Trust on local terms and conditions remains low. Second, that a variety of strategies are being adopted by Trust management to achieve their goal of having all staff on Trust conditions. These range from a gradual movement, through a phased group by group strategy to the 'big bang' strategy which attempts to move all staff to Trust conditions in a single move.

The main barrier to moving staff to Trust conditions is that staff transferring from directly managed units have the right to retain their previous Whitley based conditions and bargaining rights. The Department of Health advised that the Transfer of Undertakings (Protection of Employment) Regulations 1981 applied, and subsequent Tribunal cases have verified that these regulations do apply to the public sector. Trusts could, however, establish new terms and conditions of employment and apply these to staff joining or being promoted after Trust status. Trusts generally have the objective of moving all staff onto Trust terms and conditions. However, the continued existence of nationally determined pay and conditions through either Whitley or Pay Review Bodies, means that both staff and management constantly look to these settlements which provide a backdrop minimum to anything that Trusts may decide to offer.

In moving to local pay determination, Trusts have two main options to consider. One, that pay will be determined managerially, or second, that some form of local bargaining machinery will be established. In most Trusts senior managers are on Trust terms and conditions which are not negotiated and Trusts have sought to have this key group of staff on such conditions from the beginning. For other staff, there is little evidence of attempts to have managerially determined pay for those on Trust conditions. Equally, however, there is little support for a replication of Whitley at Trust level. The preference is to establish some form of single table forum, with a reduction in the number of unions and professional associations recognised for bargaining purposes. In other Trusts staff have been grouped into a number of bargaining units, usually related to the service delivery strategy of the Trust, which is significantly less than the national Whitley arrangement. Weston, for example, has four bargaining units based on occupational groupings (clinical, medical, general support, professional and technical support).

While there is a strong desire for single table fora, this is not always practicable, particularly with regard to doctors. The BMA has a national policy of creating Local Negotiating Committees to represent medical staff solely. Separate representation for doctors has been accepted by some Trusts, such as Aberdeen Royal Hospital and RNOH. While there is a clear move to single table bargaining, in our survey there are only two examples of single union deals - both in ambulance trusts. Northumbria Ambulance balloted staff on the choice of being represented by either a staff association or an existing union. Staff voted for a union; management then invited contenders to apply. This caused the TUC unions some difficulty and they boycotted the process. APAP, on the other hand, became the sole applicant and was accepted even though they only had 9.6 percent of the staff in membership and this had risen to only 15.3 per cent 16 months later. By contrast, the other single union deal in Norfolk Ambulance is with Unison and covers 90 per cent of staff. In other Trusts, any derecognition of unions was limited to some organizations which only had a handful of members in any particular Trust.

Other changes

If progress on local pay determination has been slow, what of progress on other aspects of human resource management under the control of the Trusts? One area where Trusts were expected to make significant radical change was in alterations to skill mix. The general aim here is to maximise the amount of working time highly trained and qualified staff spend doing what they have been trained to do, and consequently to have less well qualified and lower paid staff do the more routine tasks. Healthcare assistants are one manifestation of this. This policy has been pursued at Southend, and at Weston through the General Assistant Grade. However most progress in this area has been with ancillary support services. There is little evidence that skill-mix exercises have, so far, had much impact on nurses or PAMs, and certainly not on doctors. Our findings are reinforced by those of

49

another recent survey of first and second wave Trusts, although this survey also found that 27 our of 33 Trusts were going to consider skill-mix exercises in the near future (IRS, 1993).

Containing and controlling pay costs is not just a function of pay determination procedures and the level of annual rise, but is also determined by pay structures. Criticisms of the old Whitley system included the myriad of, often overlapping, pay structures and many Trusts in their application documents wanted to effect change in this area particularly through developing a single pay structure.

There is some evidence of movement towards the single pay spine. IRS (1993) identify 8 examples of this from their 33 Trusts. We have identified 6 Trusts who have implemented single spines and 6 more who intend to do so. Yet this development is not universally welcomed by Trust personnel directors, even by those seeking to reform pay structures, because it is either seen as too difficult, or, it is seen as an end in itself which does not remove inequities in the level of reward.

Most Trusts seeking to reform pay structures, whether through the single spine or by other means, have introduced job evaluation schemes in an attempt to provide some order or logic to their pay structure. Job evaluation is also a response to the fear that equal value claims might arise from unjustifiable grading structures. The need for job evaluation has led a number of consulting firms to develop systems suitable for use in the NHS. The time to do this properly has added to the delay in moving towards new structures. Linked closely to this is the introduction of performance appraisal schemes. One feature of new pay structures is the removal of automatic annual increments and their replacement by reward systems which base increases on performance. However such changes are not widespread and in many cases confined to senior managers (IRS, 1993).

One goal virtually every Trust had set itself was to achieve harmonisation of conditions across all staff rather than the variety of often overlapping conditions stemming from the various Whitley Councils. This was not simply a tidying up administrative goal, but one presented in terms of 'the team' and a desire to eliminate unjustifiable differences. Progress on this has also been slow. In a number of Trusts RCN and RCM representatives have objected to harmonisation on the basis of current nurses and midwives conditions as this undermines their differentials with lower status groups and does not improve their conditions.

A key tenet of the human resource management approach is a change in the balance of responsibility for managing people between line and personnel management. Evidence of the development of human resource management in NHS Trusts would be of the devolution of personnel decision making to line managers coupled with evidence of personnel managers playing a more strategic policy making role. The IRS survey provides some evidence for devolution, but this is largely confined to recruitment and the majority of Trusts in their survey have only devolved some decisions to line managers. In our survey 6 Trusts had devolved day to day tasks such as discipline and recruitment to line mangers so that the personnel staff could concentrate on manpower planning, organisational development and pay determination.

It was evident from our survey that there was a concern about the preparedness of line managers for change. A range of training programmes were introduced to prepare line mangers for the new tasks they would have to undertake in the managing people area. Indeed some personnel managers reported that their workload had increased as line managers requested support for their new role.

Approaches to change

If we consider the different approaches adopted by Trust management in their attempts to establish new Trust pay and rewards strategies, we have identified in Table 3.2 three approaches: the 'big bang', the phased and staying with Whitley. Only 3 Trusts (CA, NAS, WDMH) have adopted the 'big bang' method of introducing new terms and conditions for Trust staff from day one of Trust status. The right of staff to retain their Whitley conditions somewhat diluted the effect of the explosion.

The majority of Trusts in our survey adopted a phased approach. This was either by staff group or by introducing new procedures before making substantive changes. The staff group approach is illuminating when we come to consider barriers to change in the NHS. The first group for new contracts is always the senior mangers who have Trust contracts based on individual contracts, no collective bargaining and performance related pay. The next group is usually the 'hotel services' staff, a group which is somewhat depleted from pre-trust days by the impact of Compulsory Competitive Tendering. Then follow maintenance staff, estates staff and administrative and clerical staff. Only after this are PAMs, nurses and finally doctors tackled.

The procedures first approach involves the introduction of job evaluation and skill mix exercises to underpin new substantive changes in remuneration packages, and may also be combined with the group by group phasing discussed above. This strategy of staged and incremental change being pursued in human resource management ties in with strategies of an incremental pattern of change within professionalised bureaucracies identified elsewhere (Pettigrew et al., 1992).

Finally some trusts have a policy of staying with Whitley in the meantime, or at least until it is abolished nationally. A variation of this is to 'wait and see' the outcome of change in the first and second eave trusts before embarking on similar exercises.

Our survey included a range of different service providers. It is clear that different types of trust are in a better position than others to change. Contrast, for example, Trusts with only one key staff group, a small number of trade unions and a limited range of services to provide, with acute general hospitals providing a wide range of services, delivered by a number of significant staff groups who are represented by an array of trade unions and staff associations. Somewhere in between lie trusts whose main service area is mental health or handicap, which have a smaller number, usually about 4, of staff groups and representatives than acute hospitals. Thus all 3 ambulance trusts in our survey have introduced a single pay spine with no incremental progression. Similarly 2 of our mental health trusts, Homewood and WDMH, have also introduced a single pay spine which although more complex than in the ambulance trusts is much more feasible than that which would be required in the general hospital trusts.

The picture emerging from our survey and confirmed by the IRS (1993) survey is that change in the human resource management area in NHS Trusts has not been as rapid or as widespread as anticipated in 1991. This particularly applies to local pay determination, but also applies to a range of human resource management practices. If human resource management is defined by the coherent integration of a range of practices with each other and with the business strategy of the organisation, then there is little evidence of it being practised in NHS Trusts. The picture, however, is uneven, with some Trusts making quite rapid and radical changes, such as our 3 ambulance trusts, but other moving much more slowly, and other again hardly at all.

Understanding change: professionals in the NHS

Given these findings about slow and uneven movement on the key changes in employment relations in NHS Trusts, we now attempt to understand this situation in the light of our earlier discussion about 'conformist and deviant innovator' strategies for NHS personnel managers. We have suggested that the most likely approach to managing change which NHS personnel managers would adopt would be the 'conformist innovator'. This, as we have seen, requires personnel managers to commit themselves to organisational goals and to ally themselves with senior managers who are key in determining these. This, however, is not straight forward in an NHS context.

If the NHS has some specific culture, then a key feature of this is the role played by the various groups of professional workers within it. In terms of managing professional employees there has been great stress by professionals themselves that they should not be managed by people outside their particular profession. Or as Nelson (1989, p. 132) put it 'there is also a tendency among many professionals to hold that the only group that can legitimately change what a profession does is that profession itself'. Strong and Robinson (1990) argue that this 'syndicalist' approach to medical organisation was reflected in the management of the NHS up to and including the 1974 reorganisation. 'Accountants would manage accountants, doctors would manage doctors, nurses would manage nurses, then, through consultation and committees the sum of things would be co-ordinated' (p. 18).

It was this notion and practice of consensus management that was challenged by the Griffiths' report (1983) and the introduction of general management into the NHS in the following year. Strong and Robinson see this as a decisive break with the old syndicalist system and the power of the professions. In particular they argue that the position of the nursing profession was decisively weakened, despite their protests at the time.

While some success for general managers has been acknowledged, Harrison et al., (1992) believe the that the Conservative government had 'underestimated the power of doctors to resist challenges to their traditional way of doing things' (p. 2), especially at the local level. The power of doctors is seen to operate at two levels. At the macro-level, through the British Medical Association and the Royal Colleges they shape national health policy. At the micro-level their decisions about patient care, despite their (often considerable) resource implications are unlikely to be challenged by either managers or other occupational groups within the NHS. Harrison et al. further argue that the power of doctors is reinforced by cultural factors, such as the high social status and respect they enjoy from the general public, and within the health service from other occupational groups. 'These cultural factors have helped doctors to achieve their immediate personal aims and preserve their local autonomy with a minimum of overt conflict' (p. 18).

They go further and after reviewing the impact of general management after 1984 argue that 'while the management culture has visibly shifted, there has been no concomitant shift on the medical side. General management has not even challenged the medical domain never mind having succeeded in making significant inroads into it' (p. 100).

They suggest that the 1990s reforms indicate some weakening of macro medical power, but the local micro power continues to hold up well. However, they argue that *Working for Patients* puts some additional levers of power and persuasion into managers' hands which give some potential to rein in doctors clinical autonomy. But general management has been a 'crucial step in increasing the authority of managers over nurses and other professional groups, except for doctors' (p. 147).

Human resource managers' strategies

This battle for power with the NHS has significant implications for human resource managers attempting to pursue 'conformist innovator' strategies. There is no clear cut single objective of organisational success, and even more so, there is no single clear cut group of managerial colleagues with whom to align. While general managers' position has grown since their introduction, and probably especially since 1991, their position is by no means dominant. Harrison et al. (1992) argue that they suffer from one enormous drawback-they are 'seen as agents of the government in the way that doctors, nurses and other service provided are not' (p. 148). In short they are not seen as being part of the NHS tribal club. This clearly poses problems for human resource managers seeking to ally with general managers. To underscore this point Pettigrew et al. (1992) have identified managers who enjoy good relationships with clinicians, and hospitals where managers and doctors understand each others problems, as high scorers on the scale of successful change. Where there is conflict, change is less likely.

One possible response by doctors to the incursions of general management might be for them to take over general management positions themselves as an attempt to limit central government interference and to maximise local autonomy. Even if this were to be the case, it poses severe problems for human resource managers who are not really needed as part of a doctors' strategy to limit central interference in what they do.

Yet perhaps the best opportunity NHS personnel mangers have in contributing to change in Trusts is when they do act in alliance with powerful managers, be they Trust chief executives or perhaps, more rarely clinical directors. If there is to be some form of organizational culture change in the NHS, personnel managers may not be the initiators of it, but allied with powerful general mangers they may be able to challenge the culture of the professions, especially medicine. Williams et al (1989) have found that in other settings personnel managers rarely initiate significant cultural change, but they can have an important role in helping to implement it efficiently through training and communications. But success in pursuing such a strategy would imply, inter alia, that personnel directors were on the 5 person Trusts Executive Board. However, various pieces of research indicate that this is not universally the case. Guest and Peccei (1992) found that personnel representation at board level, at 65 per cent, was less likely in Trusts than in DMUs. In our sample not all personnel directors were Board members and the IRS (1993) found a similar picture with personnel losing out to the Director of Operations in a number of Trusts. Guest and Peccei's (1992) research suggests that board representation does matter and 'where personnel is formally represented on the Board with the executive team, the personnel department tends to be significantly more influential' (p. 43).

But in NHS Trusts such a strategy for human resource managers is fraught with dangers. The change being sought by chief executives, perhaps especially those brought in from outside the NHS, may be resisted by senior professionals especially from medicine and nursing. There will be resistance from professional organisations and trade unions to policies which challenge their power and their definition of professional care. In such an environment many NHS personnel staff may seek to play a mediating role between the competing champions of NHS objectives, or continuing to play a 'contracts managers' role of deploying systems and procedures.

There is evidence of this ambiguity in our survey. Bradford was at the forefront of change in 1991, but the pace of innovation slowed markedly when the first chief executive left after failing to effect radical change quickly. West Dorset General was also held to be an exemplar in the initial stages of Trusts, but plans for change floundered under pressure from other line managers. In other Trusts opposition from professional bodies and trade unions forced modifications or a change of pace. Weston conceded a professional and technical bargaining unit when the PAMs objected to being lumped in with nurses. COHSE was able to put back some of the minimising of the trade union role at Homewood and in the West Dorset Trusts.

The locus of the most far reaching and significant change in employment relations, that we have identified is in ambulance Trusts. Jobs have been radically restructured, unions effectively sidelined, local managerial pay determination introduced, and incremental pay abolished. In these Trusts the driving force for change was the chief executive. Personnel managers may have played a role, but it was very much a supportive one. In ambulance Trusts there was a clear objective about the goal and no organised professional groups to block change or modify it to their ends. And no doubt the view expressed by one chief officer that the ambulance service 'was a tightly disciplined, uniformed single service, run by tough management, fairly autonomous from the NHS' contributed to the possibility of effecting change quickly in these Trusts.

In other Trusts where employment relationships are being restructured there is evidence of strong alliances between chief executives and personnel directors, between line management and human resource management. These human resource directors are more likely to be members of executive boards and to fulfil the criteria for the relationship between line and personnel management set out earlier by Caines. In short in Trusts where change has been more significant and introduced more quickly, human resource directors match most of the criteria of the conformist innovator. But the barriers to change are also significant. If the conformist innovator needs a successful alliance with other senior managers in order to be successful, the NHS Trusts are a risky place to seek such alliances as it is by no means clear who is going to win the battle between managerialism and professionalism.

However, the recent evidence from IRS and ourselves suggests that innovation is not widespread and certainly does not live up to the expectation of 1991. While some evidence for the existence of 'conformist innovators' does exist, we must conclude that the dominant form of personnel management in the NHS remains the 'contracts manager'.

References

Armstrong, P. (1991), 'Limits and possibilities for HRM in an age of management accountancy', in Storey, J. (ed) *New Perspectives on Human Resource Management*, Routledge, London.

Briscoe, S. (1991), 'Meeting The Training Needs of NHS Personnel Specialists', *Personnel Management*, July, pp. 41-45.

Bryson, C., Jackson, M. and Leopold, J. (1993), *Self Determination in NHS Trusts: Impact on Industrial Relations and Human Resources Management*, University of Stirling, Stirling.

Caines, E, (1992), 'Health Service Needs a Massive Push on Productivity', *Personnel Plus*, October, p. 12.

Caines, E. (1993), 'Amputation is Crucial to the Patient's Health', *Guardian*, 12 May, p. 20.

Davies, P. (1993), 'Beware of Outside Agitators', *Health Services Journal*, 10 June, p. 24.

Department of Employment (1988), *Employment for the 1990s*, HMSO Cmd. 540, London.

Department of Health & Social Services (1983), *Report of the NHS Management Inquiry*, (Griffiths Report), HMSO, London.

Fullerton, H. and Rice, C. (1993), 'Culture Change in the NHS', *Personnel Management*, March, pp. 50-53.

Guest, D. and Peccei, R. (1992), *The Effectiveness of Personnel Management in the NHS*, NHS Management Executive, London.

Hancock, C. (1992), 'Expectation of Management', *Senior Nurse*, 12.3, pp. 4-7.

Harrison, S., Hunter, D. J., Marnoch, G. and Pollitt, C. (1992), *Just Managing: Power and Culture in the National Health Service*, Macmillan, Basingstoke.

Hodges, C. (1991), 'Metamorphosis in the NHS: The Personnel Implications of Trust Status', *Personnel Management*, April.

Hugman, R. (1991), *Power in Caring Professions*, Macmillan, Basingstoke.

Industrial Relations Services (1993), 'Local Bargaining in the NHS: A Survey of First and Second Wave Trusts', *IRS Employment Trends*, 537, pp. 7-16, IRS, London.

Legge, K. (1978), *Power, Innovation and Problem Solving in Personnel Management*, McGraw-Hill, Maidenhead.

Legge, K. (1991), 'Human resource management: a critical analysis', in Storey, John (ed), *New Perspectives in Human Resources Management*, Routledge, London.

Leopold, J.and Beaumont, P. (1985), 'Personnel Officers in the NHS in Scotland: development and change in the 1970s', *Public Administration*, 63.2, pp. 219-226.

Leopold, J. and Beaumont, P. (1986), 'Pay bargaining and management strategy in the NHS', *Industrial Relations Journal*, 17.1, pp. 32-45.

Lyall, J. (1991), 'Top Managers - The NHS Must Grow Its Own', *Health Manpower Management,* 17.2, pp. 4-5.

McCarthy, L. (1976), *Making Whitley Work*, DHSS, London.

Munro, M. (1992), 'The Expert Plus Role of Personnel Advisers in An NHS Trust', *Health Manpower Management*, 18.2, pp. 22-24.

Nelson, M. J., (1989), *Managing Health Professionals*, Chapman and Hall, London.

Pettigrew, A., Fairlie, E. and McKee, L. (1992), *Shaping & Strategic Change,* Sage: London.

Raelin, J. (1985), *The Clash of Cultures: Managers and Professionals*, Harvard University Press, Cambridge.

Salaman, G. (ed) (1992), *Human Resource Strategies*, Sage, London.

Spry, C. and Cainnes, E. (1991), 'Big Bang Hits The Health Service', *Personnel Management*, January, pp. 23-72.

Storey, J. (ed.), (1991), *New Perspectives on Human Resource Management*, Routledge, London.

Storey, J. (1992), *Development in the Management of Human Resources*, Blackwell, Oxford.

Strong, P. and Robinson, J. (1991), *The NHS Under New Management*, Open University Press, Milton Keynes.

Torrington, D. (1991), 'Human Resource Management and the Personnel Function', in Storey, John (ed), *New Perspectives on Human Resource Management,* Routledge, London.

TUC Health Services Committee (1982), *Improving Industrial Relations in the National Health Service*, TUC, London.

Tyson, S. and Fell, A. (1986), *Evaluating the Personnel Function*, Hutchinson, London.

Williams, A and Dobson, P. and Walters, M. (1989), *Changing Culture*, Institute of Personnel Management, London.

4 A management role for the general practitioner?

Sheila Greenfield and Amanda Nayak

Introduction

The role, duties and technical support of general practitioners have changed significantly in the last twenty years. The traditional single-handed doctor has now largely given way to a more complex structure of group practices typically ranging from six to fifteen personnel. Doctors, nurses and receptionists have become teams of professionals offering a wide range of services integrated with hospitals, health visitors and social workers (Morrell, 1991; Hasler, 1992). Practices therefore are now faced with the problems of providing an efficient and effective service whilst meeting the professional and personal aspirations of a highly skilled, idiosyncratic workforce.

As the running of general practices became more complex, a process of reorganisation has been taking place leading to an increased emphasis upon more formalised and business like methods. These developments have included the employment of practice managers to assist with management and administration (Pringle, 1991) and the trend towards computerisation (Middleton, 1990). These were voluntary developments on the part of practices, and general practitioners were able to choose the extent to which they embraced such developments.

A radical change however came in the shape of the new contract which was introduced on the 1st April 1990 (Department of Health, 1989b) following Government reports in the late Eighties (Secretaries of State 1987; Department of Health, 1989a). The stated aim of the new contract was to make general practices more businesslike and improve the services offered to patients. It defined the duties and range of services provided by general practitioners in a more formal way, changed the way doctors are remunerated and emphasised the role of the doctor in preventing as well as treating illness. A year later general practices with a list size of 11,000 patients were also given the opportunity to become budget holders, controlling budgets delegated to them for the purchase of the health care needs of their patients. This opportunity has gradually been extended to include smaller practices.

An important impact of these changes has been on practice finance and administration. The requirements of the new contract now mean that all general practices have to be run on business lines, whether doctors like it or not, both in order to fulfil certain stated requirements and to maintain practice income. For all practices therefore this has meant the introduction of additional administrative, negotiating, information technology and financial skills not provided during medical training (Dean, 1989) or previously experienced by doctors in running a practice.

But how do general practitioners feel about taking on a management role? To what extent do they need training in financial and management skills to enable them to cope with their changed role? What specific subject areas are most crucial and what training methods are most appropriate for teaching both practising and future general practitioners these skills?

This paper sets out to describe general practitioners' responses to the management role which has been imposed on them and their perceptions of training needs in this area. It will focus on:

1 general practitioners' attitudes to the management role.
2 their perceptions of business training needs before the new contract (i.e. while they were anticipating change and not actually having to put business skills into practice).
3 their practical response to the new contract in terms of changes they had to make to their practices.
4 their perceptions of business training needs after the new contract.

Method

Information about attitudes and training needs was obtained from two separate research studies:

1 Responses from 168 general practitioners who replied to a postal questionnaire sent to all the 307 general practitioners listed as Course Organisers or Regional Advisers in General Practice in the fifteen Regional Health Authorities in England and Wales. (Greenfield and Nayak, 1992) The questionnaire, which was sent out one year before the introduction of the new contract asked general practitioners:

(a) the extent to which they felt there was a need for formal training in financial and practice management skills.

(b) in which subject areas training was needed.

(c) at what career stage financial and practice management skills should be taught.

(d) the extent of their knowledge of locally based courses in financial and practice management skills.

2 Responses given by a random sample of 251 general practices to a postal questionnaire sent out one year after the introduction of the new contract which asked about the impact of the new contract on their business methods and information needs. (Greenfield et al., 1991).

Results

General practitioners' attitudes towards the management role

Responses to the questionnaire showed that general practitioners did not view the prospect of having to adopt business methods at all positively. They felt first and foremost that this was *not part of their professional role*:

> Doctors are not trained to be managers and even if one employed suitable managers I feel that as a Co-director of one's company one must have an insight and knowledge to run an efficient ship. I do not *want* to spend time doing this when my skills could be used for practical benefit...

> If I had wanted to become a businessman I would have gone into commerce. If I wanted to make money I would move over into antiques or real estate and double my income overnight. I spent six hard years qualifying and did four house jobs to become a GP and treat patients.

> I went into this to practice medicine and not to be an accountant.

Other factors mentioned were *the amount of time involved*:

> Look mate! I want to spend time with patients trying to be a bit of help occasionally. I am not an accountant nor do I want to waste time on administration.

> ...an inordinate amount of time will be required and be taken away from the professional work of medicine.

the anticipated *increase in workload* that would ensue:

> more and more paperwork.
> I consider I have enough to do.
> We do not need any more adrninistrative tasks with paperwork spin offs.

and a most important consideration *lack of appropriate skills*:

> I am a doctor not a manager - I have had no management training .
> I do not feel that my medical training has given me the management skills to undertake this type of work.
> I was trained as a doctor not an accountant. Patients are more important than paper.

Perceptions of financial and management skills training needs before the new contract

Need for formal training An overwhelming majority of the 168 general practitioners who replied to the pre-contract questionnaire said that there was a need for formal training in both financial skills, (162:96 per cent) and in practice management skills. (163:97 per cent).

Subject areas A wide range of subject areas were mentioned, reflecting the variety of skills involved in running a general practice. 150 general practitioners listed at least one subject area (with a mean of 3.3 per respondent) under the heading 'financial skills', and 27 different subjects were mentioned in total (Table 4.1). The four financial subject areas most often mentioned as requiring formal training were accounts (47.3 per cent), tax (40.6 per cent), budgeting (34.6 per cent) and bookkeeping (24.6 per cent). For Practice Management Skills, 135 general practitioners listed at least one subject area, (with a mean of 4.3 per respondent) and 51 were mentioned altogether (Table 4.2). The areas causing most concem were the employment of staff (58.5 per cent), staff relationships (40.0 per cent), management theory (22.0 per cent) and managing change (20.7 per cent).

In both of these areas there was a wide diversity of perceived need, each practitioner having his own individual needs, for example 8.1 per cent requested training in recall systems whereas only 0.7 per cent required training in clinical management. A few of those who felt there was a need for training did not specify particular topics, and it is conjectured that this is because they were unsure which particular subject areas were required.

When training should take place General practitioners were asked to state at what stages of the medical career (undergraduate level, Vocational Training Scheme, in practice as a general practitioner) formal training should take place. Their replies indicated that the Vocational Training Sceme was seen to be the most appropriate place for training but many general practitioners saw training as an ongoing process beginning during undergraduate education and continuing throughout a doctor's career (Table 4.3).

Courses run in the respondents' locality When asked to describe any courses in financial skills and practice management that had taken place in their own locality during the last two years approximately 40 per cent of respondents said that in their Regions either there were no courses or they were unaware of the provision that existed. (Table 4.4).

Courses covering a total of 20 different subject areas were listed under the heading of Financial Skills (Table 4.5). Practice Accounts (27.6 per cent), Practice Finance (27.4 per cent) and the Red Book[1] (20.5 per cent) were mentioned most often. Fifty-one different practice management subject areas were listed showing the wide variety of topics that this heading embraces (Table 4.6). The greatest provision of courses appeared to be those dealing with the nature of practice management (59.5 per cent), staff management (24.4 per cent), and managing change (19.1 per cent). The wide variety of courses and the variability within Regions demonstrates the unco-ordinated approach to management training which existed before the introduction of the new contract.

The New Contract: administrative changes General Practitioners, albeit reluctantly, had to make administrative changes in their practices to cope with the demands of the new contract. These were many and varied, and had resulted in an increase in practices' paperwork and overall workload. As can be seen from Table 4.7 twenty-two different administrative changes were mentioned; whilst most practices had made several changes, some it appeared had undergone a complete catharsis:

> the practice has completely undergone a transformation both to be able to cope with the new contract and because scarcely any recording either on patients or finance was carried out previously.

The most fundamental and expensive change was 'employed more staff or existing staff for longer hours' mentioned by 51.8 per cent. Acquiring or updating computer facilities was also commonplace. Some form of record keeping change had also been introduced by 43.5 per cent of practices (i.e. keeping either for the first time, or in a more detailed manner, records of doctor/patient encounters, referrals and patient statistics).

Computerisation 71.7 per cent of practices said they had a computer. In most case (81.4 per cent) this had been introduced within the last four years and over half (56.8 per cent) said they had computerised since the beginning of 1989 i.e. in the twelve months directly prior to the introduction of the new contract (Table 4.8). This shows a significant increase just prior to the implementation of the contract.

Just over half of computerised practices (55 per cent) had also subsequently gone on to further develop their computer system by buying extra terminals or software. Nearly two thirds of practices (64.4 per cent) however reported having had problems with their computers and it was apparent that on the whole computers were used only for basic functions such as age-sex registers (97.7 per cent), repeat prescriptions (86.6 per cent, prescribing (73.8 per cent) and morbidity records (70.0 per cent).

Practice managers Although it had been expected that the number of Practice Managers would increase due to the new contract requirements, this was not borne out by the study data. 75.7 per cent of the study practices employed a Practice Manager, a not dissimilar proportion to those which used cmputer, however a different pattern of adoption over time had emerged. The figures showed a steady increase over the previous ten years as practices have expanded and systems have become more complex. This process however accelerated slightly in the year of the contract with 20.0 per cent of practices employing a practice manager for the first time but this was not as dramatic as the change in computer use. (Table 4.9).

Record keeping changes Most practices had made significant record keeping changes in order to make claims under the new contract (Table 4.10). The greatest increases occurred in areas where the information was previously less important but is now needed to make claims or monitor patients' use of resources i.e. 'the number of patients referred to hospital' (from 40.8 to 89.5 per cent), 'hospital services provided to patients' (from 17.2 to 61.8 per cent) and 'minor operations performed in the surgery' (from 29.4 to 80.9 per cent). This Table also demonstrates that an increasing number of practices were developing systems to record the use of their resources (e.g. the number of consultations made by each doctor and practice nurse). In all cases where the contract required more information in order for claims to be made the number of practices keeping appropriate records had increased.

The New Contract: advice and training received

Family Health Service Authorities Family Health Service Authorities (FHSAs) are responsible for planning and managing services in each area, including the level and quality of provision. They must also monitor and enforce standards. It is this body which keeps records of services provided by local clinics, doctors and nurses visiting schools and general practitioners and it is to this body that claims for payment are sent. Since the implementation of the new contract FHSAs, in addition to their role asco-ordinators of primary health care services have been requird to be responsible for introducing 'indicative prescribing budgets for general practitioners; GP practice budgets for certain practices; medical audit; information technology to facilitate monitoring of GP prescribing and referral rates' (Department of Health, 1989c).

FHSAs did appear to have taken on an advisory role in 1989-90 in regard to the new contract as most practices had received some help from them, (Table 4.11), in the form of general newsletters, leaflets and bulletins to 35.4 per cent of respondents. Meetings, workshops and seminars were attended by 26.7 per cent, 2 per cent had received visits from FHSA personnel and 5.6 per cent obtained advice by telephone.

Some practices were critical of their FHSA, 6 per cent received very little advice and an additional 5.2 per cent felt that the FHSA did not know the answers to problems or provided advice too late. This was however at a time when the FHSA were themselves having to adapt to new administrative demands. Resources were stretched and information was at a premium. One general practitioner summarised the situation as 'The blind leading the blind'.

Other Advisors The FHSA was not the only advisor, other sources of advice and training had been used by over half (55.0per cent) of respondents (Table 4.12). 13.9 per cent had referred to press or journal articles and 8.8 per cent had used the General Medical Services Council Survival Guide (GMSC, 1990). In all, 138 respondents mentioned a wide variety of different sources of advice that they had used, but 48 (19.1 per cent) respondents did not answer the question and 65 (25.9 per cent) used no additional advice or training. When asked in what way training and advice had not been useful there were very few responses (Table 4.13).

After the New Contract: Perceived Training Needs
General practitioners indicated that there were several areas of management which they found difficult, in particular financial planning (50.2 per cent) (Table 4.14). It is surprising in the light of this and responses to the previous questionnaire that few respondents felt that they had training needs (Table 4.15).

Discussion
The anticipated introduction of the new contract with all that this implied in terms of financial and management skills forced general practitioners to think more about a facet of their practices that had not hitherto been a priority for most family doctors. General Practitioners expressed great concern about having to become 'managers' at all, both in terms of what they felt their professional role should be (Laughlin et al., 1992), how they would actually cope with the practicalities and the potentially harmful effects on workload and patient care which might result.

That there was a very real problem in practical terms was demonstrated by the fact that prior to the new contract in the survey practices there had been a wide disparity in the records kept by doctors with regard to both practice activities and accounting records. The most efficient practices kept information on all aspects of the practice, they also monitored their income and expenditure and produced budgets. But it appeared that some practices kept hardly any records at all either of income or patient details other than those required for patient notes.

Nearly all general practitioners had had to make changes in the way their practices were organised, in particular in terms of equipment and staffing to assist them with increased record keeping, but for some practices the impact of the enforced changes was greater than for others. As shown elsewhere (Bain, 1991a; 1991b; Hannay et al. 1992a; 1992b) this had resulted in an increased workload.

Although a year after the new contract, very few doctors responded positively, some did feel that the situation in their practices had improved as a result of the changes they had made:

> Much better all round, better working environment and control over patients seen.
> We are just beginning to reap the benefits after nine months of hard work.

But it was clear that for most the efforts they had had to make were causing considerable strain and the fears they had expressed about the effect on workload and patient care had been realised.

> Extra work - running like hell to stay in the same place, senior partner determined on early retirement, practice manager longing for retirement, one receptionist leaving. Basically we are getting by, but it is an effort and mostly not patient oriented.

> Mayhem in working area - greater volume of paperwork in ever increasing loads - greater need for staff counselling due to increased work load. Patients see me less - more orientation towards business attitudes and I feel I am becoming less a doctor and getting away from the principles and fundamental feelings.

Despite the fact they were obviously struggling, in contrast to the need for further training in a wide range of financial and management skills expressed by the majority of doctors prior to the new contract, surprisingly soon after the implimentation of the contract only just over one third expressed a need for training. This may indicate that as a whole practices now thought they knew enough about what they should do, wished to spend their time doing it and preferred to find answers to problems as they arose. It was apparent that perceived training needs were very individualistic and it may be that as a result of their experiences general practitioners had found training courses to be too general and not specific enough to meet the needs of individual practices.

Although in the post contract period doctors did not on the whole perceive a need for training, this view is somewhat contradicted by their responses to questions about a number of aspects of practice organisation. Many were experiencing computer problems and it was apparent that computer potential was not being fully exploited. Not all practices were keeping sufficient records to make all possible claims and to analyse how their resources were being used. Substantial numbers also stated they had difficulties with accounting, financial and management topics. Although practices appeared to be muddling through, if General Practitioners are going to be able to adapt fully to their new management role there is still a need for training in these fundamental areas. One-off courses however, almost certainly do not meet the underlying need for basic financial and management training.

Ongoing courses (rather than one day seminars) run by tutors with a knowledge of the specific nature of general practice would seem to be most appropriate. In this way general practitioners would be able to discuss their particular problems in each subject with tutors and fellow participants and would gain suffficient knowledge to put them in command of their practices rather than being dependant on their practice managers or accountants. Courses should be available during the vocational year and should continue as part of a general practitioner's continuing education.

FHSAs have the role of providing support for general practices. Evidence suggests (Audit Commission, 1993) that their resources are stretched, however they may be able to commission or recommend courses run by appropriately qualified professionals.

In this new climate where General Practitioners. are required to be more responsible for making economic decisions, it is clear that more resources must be channelled into effective training.

Notes

1. *National Health Service, General Medical Services statement of Fees and Allowances*. The NHS rules governing the levels of payment made to General Practitioners.

Table 4.1

Financial skills: subject areas in which general practitioners felt there was a need for formal training before the new contract (N=150)

<u>Areas mentioned by more than 10% of respondents</u>

<u>Subject</u>	<u>%</u>
Accounts	47.3
Tax	40.6
Budgeting	34.6
Bookkeeping	24.6
Red book	18.0
Financial planning	15.3
Income	14.6
Financial cost rent scheme	14.0
Use of accountant	12.6
Personal finance	12.0
Organising expenditure	12.0
Pensions	11.3
Borrowing	10.6

<u>Areas mentioned by 5-10% of respondents</u>

Cash flow, Maximising NHS income, Practice finance, Capital investment, Health service economics

<u>Areas mentioned by less than 5% of respondents</u>

Use of money, Profit sharing, Prescribing costs, Balance sheet, Relationship with banks & lenders Cost effectiveness, Claims, School fees, Section 63

*(More than one answer was given by some respondents.)

Table 4.2

Practice management skills: subject areas in which general practitioners felt there was a need for formal training before the new contract (n=135)

Areas mentioned by more than 10% of respondents

Employment of staff	58.5
Staff relationships	40.0
Management theory	22.0
Managing change	20.7
Use of time	19.2
Teamwork	17.7
Auditing performance	17.0
Planning	15.5
Delegation	14.8
Computer skills	14.0
Training staff	13.3
Buildings	11.0
Interviewing skills	10.3
Firing staff	10.3
Partnerships	10.3

Areas mentioned by 5-10% of respondents

Self management, Staff/Partner meetings FPC/Practice liaison, Contracts, Recall systems The role of the practice manager, Professional leadership, Record keeping, Motivation.

Areas mentioned by less than 5% of respondents

Decision making, Running clinics, Appointment systems, White Paper, Practice leaflets, Patient participation groups, Managing workload, Dispensing, Communication skills, Use of resource, Problem solving.

*(More than one answer was given by some respondents).

Table 4.3

Respondents views as to when formal trainlng should take place (n = 168)

	Financial Skills		Practice Management Skills	
	No.	%	No.	%
Undergraduate level	30	17.9	41	24.4
Vocational training scheme	145	86.3	132	78.6
When working as a GP	83	49.4	82	48.8

Table 4.4

Summary of courses which had taken place (N=168)

Response	Financial Skills		Practice Management Skills	
	No.	%	No.	%
At least one course	102	60.7	94	56.0
Did not know of any	16	9.5	17	10.1
No course took place	50	29.8	57	33 9

Table 4.5

**Financial skills: subject area of courses listed by general practitioners
(N=102)**

Courses mentioned by more than 10% of respondents

	%
Practice accounts	27.4
Practice finance	27.4
Red book	20.5

Courses mentioned by 5-10% of respondents

Taxation, Personal finance, Cost rent finance, Income and expenditure, Role of accountant

Courses mentioned by less than 5% of respondents

Bookkeeping, Financial management, Financial planning, Financial implications of prescribing, NHS finance, Management accounting, Balance sheet, Financial implications of White Paper, Cash flow, Savings and investment

*(More than one answer was given by some respondents)

Table 4.6

Practice management skills: subject area of courses listed by general practitioners (n=94)

Courses mentioned by more than 10% of respondents

	%
Practice management	59.5
Staff management	24.4
Managing change	19.1
Partnership	11.7

Courses mentioned by 5-10% of respondents

Audit, Premises, Time management, Teamwork, Practice reports, Legal obligations, Relationship with FPC, Setting up a clinic, Recall, Interviewing, The Role of the practice manager

Courses mentioned by less than 5% of respondents

Meetings, Computerisation, The Role of the practice nurse, Agreements, Conflict, Training, Delegation, Joining a practice, The future of general practice, Communications, NHS organization, Record keeping, Prescribing, Dealing with problem patients, Referrals, Terms of service, Contracts, Staff relationships, Equipment, Cost effective health care, Organization of care, Stress management, Setting up a practice library, Resources, Decision making, Appointment systems, The Role of the receptionist, Personal development, Leadership, Planning, Motivation, Professional representation, Standard setting, Committee work, Research, Complaints.

*(More than one answer was given by some respondents.)

Table 4.7

Changes made by general practitioners in their practices in response to the new contract (n=251)

	No	%
Employed extra staff or existing staff for longer hours	130	51.8
Computer: installed new, upgraded or expanded existing system	76	30.3
More detailed patient records	34	13.5
Collection and recording of statistics for reports, claims etc	30	12.0
Production of practice leaflet, staff contracts, claim forms	27	10.8
More efficient use of staff, redefined job descriptions, retrained	22	8.8
Allocated more time to paperwork	18	7.2
Need more space	18	7.2
Administrative changes	17	6.8
New patient questionnaire/check	17	6.8
Keeping record of hospital referrals and self referrals	16	6.4
Review of procedures on immunisation, screening etc.	12	4.8
Keeping child health surveillance register	10	4.0
Introduced practice meetings, reports	7	2.8
Now locked into target schedules	6	2.4
Changed system of sharing work load among partners	3	1.2
Business manager appointed	3	1.2
Accounts procedures - cash flow budgets	3	1.2
Wish to leave, find another post, retire, emigrate	3	1.2
Formed new partnership	2	0.8
Encounter diaries for each doctor/nurse	2	0.8
Attend more courses	2	0.8
Other	7	2.8
No specific change	5	2.0
No answer	18	7.2

Source: *Greenfield et al. (1991), p.17*

Table 4.8

When did you first install a computer in your practice? (N=180)

Year	No.	%
After 1st April 1990	38	21.3
1989 - 31.3.1990	64	35.5
1988	26	14.6
1987	18	10.0
1986	6	3.3
1985	6	3.3
1984	6	3.3
1983	2	1.1
1982	6	3.3
1980	2	1.1
Before 1980	3	1.6
No answer	3	1.6

Source: *Greenfield et al. (1991), p.9*

Table 4.9

How long has your practice employed a practice manager? (N=190)

Years	No.	%
< 1 year	38	20.0
1- < 5 years	48	25.3
5-< 10 years	44	23.2
10 years and over	58	30.5
No answer	2	1.0

Source: *Greenfield et al. (1991), p.8*

Table 4.10
Record keeping changes

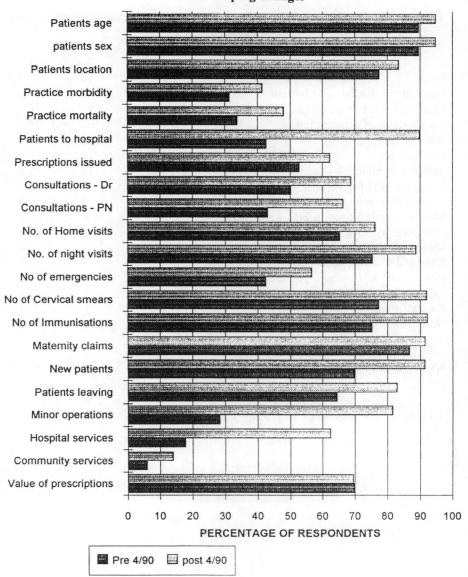

PERCENTAGE OF RESPONDENTS

■ Pre 4/90   ▩ post 4/90

Source: *Greenfield et al. (1991), p.16*

Table 4.11

Information received by doctors from FHSAs to advise them about the new contract (n=251).

	No	%
None	12	4.8
Newsletters, leaflets and bulletins	89	35.4
Meetings, workshops and seminars	67	26.7
No shortage of information	66	26.3
Very little	15	6.0
New red book	14	5.6
Telephone advice	14	5.6
Visits by FPC personnel	13	5.2
Advice on practice leaflets, recall letters, claim forms	11	4.4
Mostly showing gaps in FPC knowledge	8	3.2
Computer systems - recommendations and demonstrations	7	2.8
Directives and advice on targets	6	2.4
Received too late, appalling	5	2.0
Lists re cervical smears, geriatrics, vaccinations	4	1.6
Address of regional advisory council	2	0.8
Re staff training	1	0.4
No answer	20	8.0

*(More than one answer was given by some respondents.)

Source: *Greenfield et al. (1991), p.21*

Table 4.12

Other types of business advice, support and training received by doctors
(n=251)

	No	%
None	65	25.9
Training sessions, seminars, meetings	65	25.9
Articles in the press, journals etc	35	13.9
General medical services council survival guide	22	8.8
British Medical Association	15	6.0
LMC	12	4.8
Computer training	10	4.0
Newsletter, circulars	8	3.2
Discussions with colleagues	8	3.2
Accountants	5	2.0
Video from medical rep	3	1.2
Other	10	3.6
No answer	48	19.1

* (More than one answer was given by some respondents.

Source: *Greenfield et al. (1991), p.22*

Table 4.13

Reasons given by doctors to explain why advice and training was not useful.
(N=251)

	No	%
Needs to be more specific	19	7.5
FPC do not fully understand implications of advice DHSS	10	4.0
Communications heavily biased politically and contradictory	5	2.0
We already knew (more)	5	2.0
Arrived too late	3	1.2
Too busy to make use of it	3	1.2
Too much information	2	0.8
Press unreliable	2	0.8
Lack of phone contact with any degree of knowledge	1	0.4
No answer	201	80.0

Source: *Greenfield et al. (1991), p.22*

Table 4.14

Areas which GP's found difficult (n=251)

	No.	
Financial planning	126	50.2
Use of time	102	40.6
Management theory	100	39.8
Tax	99	39 4
Budgeting	98	39.0
Medical audit	93	37.1
Red book	69	27.5
Bookkeeping	59	23.5
Staff relationships	51	20.3
Employment of staff	44	17.5
Teamwork	27	10.8
Other	8	3.2

Source: *Greenfield et al. (1991), p.26*

Table 4.15

Areas which doctors felt they needed training/advice in after the new contract (n=251)

	No	%
None	31	12.3
Function, activities and expectations of FPC (e.g. re targets, claims, practice records, forms)	27	10.7
Accounting financial planning	23	9.2
Business/practice management skills	20	8.0
Computers/keyboard skills	19	7.6
Time/stress management	14	5.6
Negotiation of contracts, Budget management	7	2.8
Everything	8	3.2
Health promotion and minor surgery	6	2.4
Staff recruitment and reimbursement	5	2.0
Best time to retire early	5	2.0
Clinical organization/claiming	4	1.6
Data collection	4	1.6
Other (8 items)	11	6.4

* ((More than one answer was given by some respondents).

Source: *Greenfield et al. (1991), p.23*

References

Audit Commission, (1993), *Practices Make Perfect: 7he Role of the Family Health Services Authority,* HMSO.

Bain, J. (1991a), 'General practices and the new contract, I-Reactions and impact', *British Medical Journal,* 302, pp. 1183-1186.

Bain, J. (1991b), 'General practices and the new contract, II-future directions', *British Medical Journal,* 302, pp. 1247-1249.

Dean, J. (1989), 'A clean bill of financial health', *Accountancy,* pp. 172-174.

Department of Health (1989a), *Terms of Service for doctors in general practice,* London, HMSO.

Department of Health (1989b), *General Practice in the National Health Service: the 1990 Contract,* London, HMSO.

Department of Health (1989c), *Working for Patients: Implications for Family Practioner Committees Working Paper 8,* London, HMSO.

GMSC (1990), *The General Medical Services Committee Survival Guide to the New Contractual Arrangements.*

Greenfield, S., Nayak, A. and Drury, M. (1991), *Ihe Impact of Working for Patients and the 1990 Contract on General Practitioners administrative systems.* Certified Research Report 25, Certified Accountant Publications.

Greenfield, S. and Nayak, A. (1992), *Financial & Practice Management Skills: A Survey of General Practitioner Training Needs.* Departmental Working Paper. Department of Accoumting & Finance, Birmingham Business School.

Hannay, D., Usherwood, T., Platts, M. (1992a), 'Workload of general practitioners before and after the new contract', *British Medical Journal,* 304, pp. 615-618.

Hannay, D., Usherwood, T., Platts, M. (1992b), 'Practice organisation before and after the new contract', *British Journal of General Practice,* 42, pp. 517-520.

Hasler, J. (1992), 'The primary health care team: history and contractual farces', *British Medical Journal,* 305, pp. 232-234.

Laughlin, R., Broadbent, J., Shearn, D. (1992), 'Recent Financial and Accountability Changes in General Practice: An Unhealthy Intrusion into Medical Autonomy', *Financial Accountability and Management* 8, pp. 129-148.

Middleton, J. (1990), 'How will the White Paper change General Practice', *Modern Medicine,* pp.39-45.

Morrell, D. C. (1991), 'Role of research in development of organisation and structure of general practice', *British Medical Journal,* 302, pp.1313-1316.

Pringle, M. (1991), 'The practice manager', *British Medical Journal,* 303, pp. 146-147.

Secretaries of State for Social Services (1987), *Promoting Better Health* (CM249) London, HMSO.

5 'Practices' and market-control: work experiences of doctors, scientists and engineers

*Terry McNulty, Richard Whittington
and Richard Whipp*

Introduction

Increasingly, the work activities of professionals and knowledge-workers are subject to market-control. The creation of 'internal markets' and the process of contracting-out mean that work is now often managed on a customer-contractor basis (Halal et al., 1993; Whittington, 1992; Yorke, 1990; Smith, 1989; Savage et al., 1988; Sveiby and Lloyd, 1987; Torrington and McKay, 1986) This chapter discusses implications of market-control for the work of doctors in UK National Health Service (NHS) hospitals as well as scientists and engineers in industrial Research & Development (R&D) laboratories. The findings are relevant to broader debates about the market control of organizations and activities (Macintyre, 1990; Keat, 1991) as well as the work experience in contemporary market economies (Lane, 1991).

The chapter uses the concept of 'practice' (Macintyre 1990) in preference to the established concepts and orthodox language offered by the sociology of the professions (Abbott, 1988). Medicine, engineering and science are treated as practices. Macintyre (1990) defined a practice, as an activity, guided by collectively established 'standards of excellence' which those individuals engaged with a practice endeavour to adhere to and enhance. In the process of doing so they realise 'internal goods'. For Macintyre (1990) and Keat (1991) the realisation of internal goods and enhancement of practice standards of excellence can be undermined by subjecting a practice to market forces. Following this argument, the chapter asks whether the creation of the NHS internal market (Dept of Health, 1989) and market-control of industrial R&D (Whittington, 1992) are damaging to the practices of medicine, engineering and science?

The question is addressed using data collected during the intensive study of four NHS hospitals and four Research and Development (R&D) laboratories. Initially, the chapter describes those work experiences of doctors, engineers and scientist which suggest that practices are vulnerable to market control. However, the chapter then goes on to describe experiences of doctors, scientists and engineers which suggest that practices are enhanced by market relations. These positive experiences indicate that the implications for practices of market relations are not as adverse and detrimental as existing practices literature argues.

Relations between practices and markets are not so clear-cut that practices should be viewed as necessarily either vulnerable or invulnerable to market pressures. The chapter concludes by suggesting that an intellectual challenge for the future is identifying contingencies in the complex web of relationships between practices, organizations and markets. Pointers to the direction of further analysis are offered by the suggestion that the implications for practices of market-control depends on the character of the market which individuals engaged in practices are exposed to, approaches within organisations to managing individuals engaged in practices and each individual's work orientation and expectations.

The chapter has five sections. The next section discusses the theoretical approach used in this chapter, and contains a fuller discussion of the concept of practice and its consideration in the light of current changes in the NHS and industrial R&D. After a brief section, describing the research study and methods, the empirical findings are discussed. The final section reports the chapter's conclusions.

Theoretical approach

The concept of 'practice'

Doctors, scientists, and engineers' experiences of working in market conditions are analyzed using the concept of 'practice' (Macintyre, 1990; Keat, 1991; Reed, 1985; 1989; 1992), rather than the language and concepts offered by the sociology of professions (Abbott, 1988; Bloor and Dawson, 1994). The dispute between Raelin (1985) and Bailyn (1985) about the professional status of engineers in industrial R&D laboratories is symptomatic of a subject plagued by a fixation on issues of definition, often at the expense of important and interesting substantive issues (Abbott, 1988). The conceptual approach offered by the sociology of professions is inadequate for studying the relations between work and markets. The professions literature is not nearly as revealing about professionals working in market conditions as it is about the plight of professionals in organizational hierarchies. The literature can be criticised for lagging behind contemporary changes (Lane, 1991; Du Gay and Salaman, 1992) in the work environment within and beyond the single firm. In contrast, discussion of the concept of practice pays attention to the role of markets in contemporary society (Keat, 1991).

Also, Abbott (1988) argued that a weakness of the professions literature is the greater concentration upon how professions are organised rather than what they do. The concern of the professions literature with the organization of occupations has diverted attention away from an individual level of analysis towards an occupational level of analysis. This may help to explain why it is that in addition to being weak in its focus upon work 'activity', the literature is inadequate in its treatment of intra and inter professional variability (Drazin, 1990). An attraction of the concept of practice is that it allows us to focus on work 'activity' rather than occupation, organization or individuals' status. Furthermore, the concept is applicable at individual and group levels of analysis without the exclusivity and definitional ambiguity associated with concepts such as 'profession' and 'professional'. Though in this chapter the concept of practice is being applied to the work of individuals often described as 'professionals', it is important to note that neither Macintyre (1990) nor Keat (1991) associate 'practices' exclusively with 'professions' or 'work'.

In this chapter medicine, science and engineering are treated as examples of a practice. Macintyre defined a practice in the following terms:

.... human activity through which goods internal to that form of activity are realised in the course of trying to achieve those standards of excellence which are appropriate to, and partially definitive of, that form of activity, with the result that human powers to achieve excellence, and human conceptions of the ends and goods involved are systematically extended (Macintyre, 1990, p. 187).

The two defining features of a practice are first, 'internal goods' and second, collectively established 'standards of excellence'. Each of these features are now explained in more detail. For the doctor, diagnostic skill, and any resultant medical and surgical action involved in patient care may be sources of internal goods. Similarly, for scientists and engineers, analytical skill, and expertise contained within the development of new formulae, processes and products are potential sources of internal goods. These goods are 'internal' because they can only be recognised and described with reference to the activity and identified by participation in it. They are different from 'external goods', examples of which are prestige, status and money. Unlike internal goods, external goods are only 'contingently attached' to a practice. They can be achieved in ways other than engaging in a particular practice. When people participate in a practice primarily for external goods, the standards of excellence of that practice become valued only instrumentally, not intrinsically as in the case of internal goods (Keat, 1991). In addition, external goods are relatively exclusive in comparison to internal goods. In competition for external goods there are typically winners and losers, whereas internal goods resulting from competition to excel, have a capability to be for the good of the whole community involved in a particular practice. The second defining feature of a practice are the collectively established standards of excellence. To enter into a practice is to accept the authority of existing standards.

Relationships with predecessors and peers are bounded by these standards. The standards of excellence are dynamic because what is involved in a practice is a process of 'critical reflection' on existing goals and standards (Keat, 1991). This process of reproduction is key in distinguishing a practice from a set of techniques which a practice typically incorporates. Part of the distinctiveness of a practice stems from the ways in which perceptions of ends and internal goods (which technical skills help to achieve) are 'transformed' and 'enriched' by extensions of capabilities and concern for internal goods (Macintyre, 1990, p. 193). It is possible to link the concept of practice with the professions literature. First, standards of excellence appear to correspond closely to 'entry controls', 'education programmes' and 'codes of conduct' associated with models of the professionalised occupation (Watson, 1987). Second, Larsen (1977) and Ritti (1971) have described the success enjoyed by particular 'occupations' in defining the relevance of their standards to institutional needs.

Practitioner, organisation and market relations

Having described a practice, the three-way set of relationships (figure 5.1) help to explain how organisations and markets each create pressures for an individual, labelled 'practitioner', engaged in a practice. These pressures can undermine the realisation of internal goods and advancement of a practice's standards of excellence (Macintyre, 1990; Keat 1991). Following Macintyre (1990) and Keat (1991), the expectation is that pressures upon doctors, scientists and engineers will intensify as NHS hospitals and industrial R&D labs are subjected to greater market control.

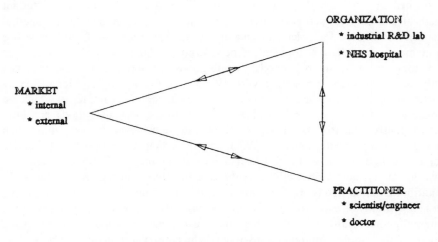

Figure 5.1   Practitioner, market, organization relationship

Practitioner and organization

Within the professions literature the concept of autonomy has traditionally been used to explain the conflict between scientists, engineers, doctors and their employing institutions (Ritti, 1971; Bailyn, 1985; Harrison, 1988). Macintyre (1990) and Keat (1991) explain conflict by reference to the paradoxical relationship between practices and organizations. For example, physics, engineering and medicine are examples of practices which Macintyre (1990) would suggest need to be sustained by institutions such as laboratories, universities and hospitals in order to survive. However, this is an uneasy coexistence because practices are vulnerable to institutions' need to generate money and other resources (external goods). These external goods can be 'damaging' to a practice as the pursuit of external goods may become an end in itself. Institutions' structure of power and reward may subvert practice rules and standards rather than maintain them. Also, the system of external rewards may diverge sufficiently from evaluations of contributions to a practice that internal goods do not provide sufficient motivation for practice participants (Keat, 1991, p. 222).

Practitioner and market

Keat (1991) argues that markets, as a domain within which producers compete with each other to sell their goods and services, are unfavourable for the 'integrity of practices' for the following reasons. Market competition is oriented to the achievement of external goods at the expense of internal goods. Markets operate on a reward structure which is 'exclusive' and discourages the sharing of ideas amongst practice participants working in competing organizations. Market success, driven by the satisfaction of potential consumers, may serve to undermine practice standards as consumers rather than producers determine what is 'good' and 'what is bad'. In other words, consumers 'wants' 'wishes' or 'preferences' take priority over producers 'ideals' (Keat, 1991, p. 223).

Organization and market: The market control of hospitals and industrial R&D laboratories.

Since the 1970s, industrial R&D in the United Kingdom has increasingly shifted on to a market control basis, leading to 'R&D professionals' (Raelin, 1985) working as consultants externally or on a customer-contractor principle internally (Whittington, 1992). Similarly, the creation of the NHS internal market (Dept of Health, 1989) has created conditions for market relations between parties responsible for purchasing health care and parties responsible for providing healthcare, with the direct relationship between the provision of care and payment for care, creating a system of incentives at the hospital level (Scrivens, 1991).

The arrows indicate that the relationships contained in figure one, are seen as interconnected and dynamic. An outcome of greater market control of these organizational contexts is that the work of doctors, engineers and scientists is increasingly subject to market pressures (Ouchi, 1980). The expectation is that these pressures upon practitioners will undermine the practices of medicine, science and engineering. Doctors, scientists and engineers, as producers/providers will lose authority as the consumer increasingly determines the form, nature and quality of goods and services (Keat, 1991). The 'producer culture' will be subjugated to the 'consumer culture' (Abercrombie, 1991). Seen in terms of the relationships in figure one, the potential for the practitioner to experience conflict in relationships with both the market and organization would seem to be increased.

Broadly, the anticipated effect of market pressures upon practices resembles some long-standing interpretations of the work experience in modern industrial capitalist society (Lane, 1991; Watson, 1987). Namely that the potential for practitioners to find fulfilment through work, is reduced as environmental pressures alienate those doing the work from their service/product, peers and their own labour (Watson, 1987). In the light of this discussion of practices, the remainder of the chapter is given to establishing whether doctors, scientists and engineers have experienced their practices being undermined as a consequence of NHS hospitals and industrial R&D labs becoming subject to market control.

Research study & methods

This study is based on intensive comparative analysis of eight organisations - four NHS hospitals, four industrial R&D laboratories. The research concentrated on units (eg, organised on the basis of clinical specialty or technology) within R&D labs and NHS hospitals where coping with increased market pressures had been identified by management as a critical issue.

The cases were researched by means of interviews and access to various public and internal documentation. 158 interviews have been carried out with the vast majority tape recorded and transcribed, the remainder annotated. Interviews were carried out during 1991 and 1992 with managers and practitioners (doctors in the NHS hospitals, scientists and engineers in the R&D labs). Of the four R&D labs, two (NRO and ERO) are independent research organizations and two (EngCo and ProcCo) are in-house central laboratories. Table 5.1 gives basic data on their size and sectors. All four laboratories faced intensifying market pressures. ERO, an independent lab, was formerly an industrial research association, which since the mid 1970's had been coping with major reductions in its government subsidy and a decline in membership fee income. NRO was a former government laboratory that had been privatised in the early 1980s. The EngCo laboratory was the centralised facility of a diversified engineering company, and had been facing declining corporate funding and increased reliance on the internal customer-contractor principle throughout the 1980s and early 1990s. A similar move to the customer - contractor principle and increased pressure from the operating divisions was also occurring at ProCo central laboratory, which was part of an international process industry business.

The hospitals studied are large urban acute care hospitals, outside of London, with a full range of medical and surgical services and budgets in excess of £50million. Since April 1992 Northtrust and Southtrust have been 'second-wave' NHS Trusts. EastDMU and WestDMU were 'directly managed units' (DMUs) at the time of the fieldwork but were granted NHS Trust status from April 1993.

Table 5.1

Case study organizations

Case:	Sector:	Staff:	Interviews
R&D Laboratories			
ERO	Engineering	250	23
NRO	Natural Resource	250	23
EngCo	Engineering	200	14
ProcCo	Process	1800	14
NHS Hospitals			
Northtrust	NHS	2000	15
Southtrust	NHS	2000	18
EastDMU	NHS	1500	14
WestDMU	NHS	1500	37

* Case names are, of course, pseudonyms; data are approximate for the sake of confidentiality.

Market control and the vulnerability of practices

The following discussion is based on experiences of doctors, scientists and engineers. It reveals contrasting views amongst practitioners about the implications of working in market contexts. Initially, the chapter presents those experiences which suggest 'practices' of medicine, science and engineering are vulnerable when exposed to market control. The bases of vulnerability are perceived as resulting from: reduced opportunities for engaging in long-term medical and scientific research; restricted opportunities for learning, knowledge accumulation and skill development; pressure to reduce quality standards; and threats to open communication amongst practice participants. However, by contrast this discussion is followed by data which describes positive work experiences of doctors, engineers and scientists. These positive experiences suggest that practices are not necessarily vulnerable to market forces.

Research, quality, learning, & skill development

Many technologists in EngCo and ProcCo, talked about the short- term demands of parent company divisions (their clients), threatening 'long-term technological development'. A senior engineer in EngCo remarked that:

> They (divisional clients) will pay for what they can afford, and they have a six-month time horizon and no desire to look further than their short-term product needs.

Concentration upon the short-term development needs of divisions was perceived by many as a barrier to the development of engineering and scientific technology. A Consultant Obstetrician and Gynaecologist in EastDMU spoke of difficulties of researching minimally invasive surgery techniques because of the unwillingness of purchasers to pay for what they perceive to be 'exploratory' work.

All of the scientists and engineers agreed that the major impact of laboratories being subject to market control are 'increased pressures of time and budget'. 'Utilization rate' (time charged to a client) and 'contribution' (profit from a contract) are symbols of labs' increased concern with the 'productivity' and 'profitability' of scientists and engineers. Similar changes are occurring within hospitals as concerns with productivity and efficiency are being driven by measures of 'patient throughput' and 'activity'.

Scientists and engineers widely perceived that the drive for increased productivity (coming from both within the organization, and from clients) was challenging the depth and breadth of work. Many engineers spoke of cutting down the number of tests to the bare minimum, reporting study results in less detailed reports than previously. Though keen to emphasise that 'professional standards' were being upheld, an interpretation of their experience is that practice development and the realisation of internal goods were being adversely affected by pressure to offer clients an 'engineeringly acceptable solution'. An engineer at NRO explained the phrase, which illustrates the conflict between client wants and practitioner ideals.

> (an)..area of the job which is different now is that if you are searching for a solution you could go on forever more searching for the absolute best solution. Now we say 'let us look for a solution which in engineering terms is acceptable'. One will draw the line at an engineeringly acceptable solution rather than the very best.

It was widely observed that pressures of 'time and budget' restricted opportunities for more junior engineers to learn and develop skills. At ERO it was admitted by a manager with over 20 years experience that:

> ..the younger guys do not get the insight into the entire problem that they did...because of the pressure of work, they are there to do a particular job.

At NRO, a much quoted phrase was 'black-box engineering', used widely amongst scientists and engineers to suggest that learning suffers because of commercial pressures. An engineer explained the 'black-box' dilemma in the following way:

> ...Generally, I do not have enough time to go into the technical background of what we do here...the models we use here can generally be used as 'black-box' models... I never have the time to find out why it has been done and about the techniques used to make the models.

Another scientist at NRO commented that:

> ... it does get boring if it is just a black box and you just use it and run it...In the end, you are not a programmer, you are just a computer operator, putting numbers in, seeing what it churns out and writing the report.

These comments suggest commercial pressures can lead to deskilling at the individual level which in turn appear to restrict individuals' ability to contribute to the transformation and enhancement of engineering and science as practices.

Similar concerns have been raised within the hospitals. At EastDMU, an Orthopaedic Surgeon expostulated that market pressures:

> .. might be forcing us into being skilled butchers, skilled technicians (the sort of attitude which says) 'There's a piece of meat down in (local town) that needs a knife putting in it and the metal-work inserted into the bone'... you treat him (the doctor) as a technician.

The surgeon continued:

> ....You might say: 'Isn't that your job?' Well, it's not really. You like to treat your patient as a whole, and not just the hole in the patient. You want to know about him. Does he live in the same town as you? You want to get things right for him and get things right for his family.

The Orthopaedic Consultant is worried about the conflict between his practice ideals and the 'wants' of the market. Also, that in these times of the separation of the purchasing of health care from its provision, the realisation of internal goods associated with patient care may be harder to achieve.

The views expressed above lend weight to arguments about divergence between definitions of quality held by those engaged in the practice and those which may apply in the market. Certainly the reference to 'engineeringly acceptable solutions' suggests a discrepancy between engineers' and scientists' definition of quality and that encouraged by market conditions. Similarly, amongst the majority of doctors in hospitals there is the fear that purchasers' quality standards are to be 'minimum standards' and that the emphasis will be upon the 'quantity' of care rather than the 'quality'. The following comment of a Consultant Obstetrician in SouthTrust is relevant here. He remarked that:

> ....(in obstetrics)...the purchaser has put pressure on to discharge women more quickly after they have had the baby. That pressure is a market force, because I do not think there is proven clinical benefit of this.

Who is the customer?

The majority of doctors are reluctant to confirm a changed relationship with patients to be a result of the creation of the NHS internal market. They are insistent that the 'customer' is the patient, not the purchaser of the service on behalf of the patient. At Northtrust, the comment of a doctor, with managerial responsibilities reflected the typical view:

> I do not agree that the regional agency is the customer. They are purely the purchasing agency on behalf of patients, who are the true customers - they are the ones who are receiving our services..We see the patients as our true customers.

A similar reluctance to accept customers as defined exclusively by purchasing power was revealed in the R&D laboratories too. In the two in-house laboratories, engineers and scientists were contracted for by divisions of the parent company. None the less they often felt as much obligation to the end users of divisions' products and services as to the divisions themselves. Many scientists and engineers were frustrated by restrictions put on them by divisions. At both ProcCo and EngCo, scientists and engineers complained that their corporate clients (divisions of the parent company) would refuse to let them interact with the ultimate consumers of their services, afraid that they would reveal technical insight and knowledge of which revelation was perceived not to be in the corporate interest. One EngCo engineer confessed that he was still too free with technical information in talking to customers. He commented that:

> I'm not too sure I am the right person to talk to customers. I'm quite happy to divulge information that probably shouldn't be divulged ... to say where I'm surprised that some people are going ahead with certain (EngCo) systems, and where they are leaving certain loopholes, certain black areas.

Within the NHS obvious manifestations of this contentious issue of 'who is the customer' emerge in the tension between purchasers demands and patients needs. An Orthopaedic Consultant at EastDMU said of purchasers that:

> ..we will have more of the GP fundholders putting pressure of management to move their patients through..they want their patient to jump the queue quite simply....I personally feel that I have to protect all of the people on my list, I do not intend to give priority.

The debate about 'who is the customer' illustrates conflict, for those engaged in practices, in the relationship between internal goods and external goods. In the last example, the doctor's realisation of internal goods associated with prioritising patients on the basis of clinical need, are being challenged by purchaser pressure upon the doctor to give priority, using criteria other than clinical need, in return for securing the contract. This example shows the doctor and senior members of hospital management in a dilemma presented by a market pressure. The dilemma is whether to pursue external goods, in the form of money from contracts, at the expense of internal goods which result from prioritising care according to clinical need.

Collegiate relations and communication

Competition between NHS hospitals encouraged by the internal market and NHS Trust status is perceived by some doctors as antipathetic to the collegiate culture of the medical profession. The traditional organization of doctors into medical and surgical divisions spanning a number of hospitals in the same geographical locality is perceived to be challenged by competition for patients amongst hospitals. A consequence being that competition for external goods, for example, money from contracts, is encouraged despite resultant adverse effects for service quality. East DMU Consultant surgeons in one surgical division perceived competition at the hospital level to be encouraging 'unhealthy' competition amongst consultants within the same division. This was perceived as 'breaking down' the working of the division across the localities hospitals, and challenging the future breadth and scope of service provision. Further, for some doctors, the weakening of 'professional' networks is leading to reduced opportunities for 'information exchange' with 'professional colleagues', the result of which is damaging to the advancement of the specialty in that locality. Responding to these pressures, a group of surgeons at EastDMU insisted that competition between hospitals units would not alter their freedom to refer patients to colleagues (even in a competitor hospital or clinical unit) if that was most appropriate to the needs of the patient.

There is also evidence that some doctors are unhappy about engaging in competition with colleagues purely for the achievement of money from contracts. Though it was widely accepted that doctors are a competitive breed and their practice membership encourages them to compete for reputation, it was felt that competition for money from contracts (external good) without resultant benefits in patient care (internal good) is not a sufficient motivator. A senior manager at EastDMU admitted of his consultants:

> Some of them feel that if we market successfully it can only be at someone else's expense. We are not about growing the market, we are talking about pinching other people's market share and some of them actually work in the other hospitals with which we compete... or they have pals who work there.

A Consultant Obstetrician and Gynaecologist at EastDMU confirmed this with the following comment:

> ...I would not be particularly interested in attracting additional work unless we were doing it better or had a particular skill we wanted to attract....I would hate to think there are units in the NHS that are actively going out to attract work currently being done by other units, simply in order to make their unit more successful, rather than for reasons of a better service or better care being provided.

Pressure applied by management upon scientists, engineers and doctors across all the hospitals and labs to take a more active interest in the economic consequences of their actions and an active role in the marketing of their services can also be interpreted as a threat to practices. Of particular concern to many was the time taken up by doing administration and marketing. This was perceived as time away from science, engineering and medicine. For engineers within the ERO laboratory it was said by a senior manager that:

> .. commercialisation means that they have to spend less time doing their own stuff. Commercialisation means that they have to spend 50 per cent of their time day-to-day looking after customers...whereas before, they could probably spend 100 per cent of their time doing what they wanted to do...

Some resented it because they perceived it to be a challenge to their occupational identity and purpose. For some the realisation of internal goods through these activities seemed inconceivable. Said one NRO engineer:

> ...I am interested in natural things....I am not an economics person, or a marketing person. I am not interested in money...

A West DMU consultant was equally antithetical:

> I hate this term market-place. This is medicine, it has its own language...to marketise the whole thing is an abhorrence to me....

Some engineers and scientists within the labs perceived processes of competition and selling to impinge upon their ability to be precise in all matters to do with their 'practice'. An engineer at ERO reflected on the effect of market pressures with the following comment:

> Having tried to work on a reasonably good scientific basis years ago, when you tried to be truthful and honest in everything you did ... you now have to get away from that outlook, cover up the gaps in your knowledge, put yourself over as knowing everything. It is a conflict between the way we were brought up to work - even the ethics if you like - and what is required nowadays.

These comments suggest that competitive relationships in the market place and the pursuit of external goods through contracts with clients may be capable of obstructing the collective advance of standards encouraged by open exchange of information amongst practice colleagues and clients.

Summarising, the preceding evidence supports the argument presented earlier in the chapter that the practices of engineering, medicine and science are vulnerable to market control (Macintyre, 1990; Keat, 1991). Doctors, engineers and scientists experience of market forces suggest that both the advancement of practice' standards of excellence and the realisation of internal goods are threatened by restrictions on learning opportunities; skill development; open communication; as well as challenges to professional definitions of quality.

However, challenging this argument is evidence to suggest that practices can be enhanced by market relations. Doctors, scientists and engineers have enjoyed positive market relations. These positive experiences are discussed in the next section.

Protection and enhancement of practices

Many scientists and engineers welcomed the pressures of limited time and budget resulting from client contracts believing that the relationship with the client afforded them opportunities to test and enhance their knowledge as well as display their technical competence. For many engineers and scientists, working directly with clients provided opportunities to enjoy the 'stimulus' of applied development work. Relative to 'basic' research, applied development work offers stimuli of shorter-time scales, a relatively higher turnover of work, a greater variety of problems to solve and the heightened expectation of realising a 'tangible outcome'. Finally, scientists and engineers frequently spoke of the thrill of applying technology. An engineer within the NRO laboratory said:

> Commercialism is important to me because I can see the direct effect of my work. I like to see the links between the fundamental research and the actual use of that in a real environment for a real problem.

The argument that practices are vulnerable to market forces is based, in part, on the view that the clients in the market-place possess the power to dictate to providers of products and services, both the quantity and quality of goods and services. Undoubtedly, clients purchasing engineering and scientific expertise are exercising power over those providing the expertise. A long-serving engineer at NRO said that:

> ...the customer is getting more financial control. One has to justify spending to a greater extent...You have to break things down so that the customer can see whether the test we are carrying out meet what we said we would do in the work schedule. He is also more knowledgeable. He probably comes to us with a better understanding of what he wants.

However, evidence collected in this study suggests that market relations do not necessarily make scientists and engineers deferential to clients. Clients' power, possessed either through financial resource or a greater understanding of their own needs, is not absolute. Clients do not necessarily dictate to engineers, scientists and doctors the form, nature and quality of the expertise offered. There remains within market relations scope for practitioners to shape and influence what is available to, and accepted by clients. The explanation for this has much to do with the reliance of clients on expert knowledge and advice. Increased client power is leading to greater interaction between client and practitioner. In NRO, an engineer said:

> there is a lot more toing and froing across the table both at the start of the study but throughout the study.

However, many of those interviewed for this study have experienced interaction in a positive way, speaking of relationships with clients based on collaboration and cooperation. Rather than rueing the increased power and knowledge of clients, many doctors, scientists and engineers believed these to be ingredients critical to the quality of interaction with a client.

Doctors, scientists and engineers in both sectors indicated that interactions with clients can be professionally rewarding, contributing to better work (and the realisation of internal goods) and the dynamic process by which practice standards are enhanced. A Consultant Paediatrician at NorthTrust spoke of the benefits to patient care resulting from a relationship with a knowledgeable 'purchaser' of health care. It was remarked that:

> ...we have a knowledgeable, intelligent purchaser. We have monthly information on how we are doing and a six monthly review on activity, and we can compare our practice with elsewhere. I also believe that this is slowly leading to an improvement in clinical care. It is their (the purchaser's) knowledge and grasp of the issue I like. It may mean that I do not get my way because they can produce facts and figures to support their argument but

at least I understand why I have not got my way.

Similarly a contract manager at NRO commented that:

.. I like some interaction with the client because you have got to have in mind what the client wants. Clients who are fairly familiar with what we are doing can interact with us and provide us with useful information about what they need to know.

Another said:

....I think they (clients) are beginning to understand that there is a science behind some of the things they do and that is important in helping them get their contracts completed more satisfactorily....There is more professionalism on both sides. We are prepared to listen to one another knowing that we both have good arguments. This is necessary for the success of the project.

Therefore, rather than seeing practices as automatically vulnerable to the client relationship these experiences suggest that practices can be enhanced by relationships with clients in the market-place. The likelihood of this appears to be greater when the relationship contains both clients and service providers active in the same practice. Evidence suggests that this is increasingly the case in industrial R&D. At NRO a long-serving engineer commented that:

These days we get a lot more interaction...clients are getting better qualified engineers and scientists, who have relevant backgrounds and prove to their managers that they are doing a job by asking questions and coming back to us.

There is a widespread hope amongst the majority of hospital doctors interviewed that growing numbers of general practitioners and public health doctors will be involved in the purchasing of health care. The general feeling amongst most of the hospital doctors is one of concern that many of those representatives of health authorities purchasing health care do not possess sufficient clinical expertise to be effective in this role. The following comment of a Consultant Paediatrician at NorthTrust summarised the views of the majority:

..an area that concerns me is the lack of purchasing expertise. There are well intentioned people and clever officers sitting on health authorities trying to reach decisions they know very little about. Very often General Medical Practitioners may be sitting on the health authority, or they may bring in other doctors, but it is very limited.

Using the following example, he went on to illustrate why it is such a concern:

> A recent example ...the health authority (purchaser) said 'the average length of stay for your patients is three days, so you have so many patients for so many days. This is what we will pay you'. We said 'but our average length of stay is four times longer than the figure you quoted' and we could prove it. So they did not even know the length of stay.

Amongst doctors, scientists and engineers some client relationships are not welcomed. Typically, these are relationships with a client who passive, ill-informed, lacking knowledge and financial power. An engineer who manages client contracts at NRO summed this up:

> ....the guys who do not have a clue what we are doing are hard work because you have to explain everything to them in such basic terms...they do not give us the problem in a clearly defined way.

Despite complaints about the amount of time and effort required to market and sell their services, a number admitted that continuous client contact did produce information which helps them in their work to produce a better service. This may explain why many doctors in hospitals are complaining about their lack of involvement in the process of contracting service provision with purchasers. Note the complaint of a Consultant Obstetrician and Clinical Director in NorthTrust:

> Do you know how contracts (with purchasers) are negotiated in NorthTrust? There is not a clinician in sight.

This comment is interesting because the experience of engineers and scientists in the labs is that the more significant their input into the processes of marketing and contracting services the greater control they have over what is being offered to clients. A significant observation from the R&D labs is that rather than having a lead role, marketing experts play a supportive role to engineers and scientists. Part of the explanation for this is political. In other words, the greater their involvement in client relationships the more scientists and engineers can control the work they do and who they do it for. A source of major concern within the R&D labs is the role of 'middle men', for example, marketing experts and contracting consultants. Scientists and Engineers frequently spoke of these people 'lacking understanding' in contract negotiations and 'making promises to clients' which were unrealistic.

Finally, despite the market conditions, we have found evidence that collegiate behaviour amongst professionals providing services is occurring, enabling them to enhance practices. In the R&D sector, scientists at all of the labs were involved in multi-company collaborative research and development programmes with peers from competing companies. In the NHS, there is evidence of surgeons of particular specialties discussing within clinical committees and forums policies for the management of competition. Informing these discussions is a desire to curb possible excesses of competition via 'gentlemen's agreements' on issues of patient referral, geographical boundaries and pricing.

Conclusions

This chapter has discussed implications of market control for the work of doctors in NHS Hospitals as well as scientists and engineers in industrial Research & Development (R&D) laboratories. The conclusions reflect upon the usefulness of the concept of practice for studying work in market conditions, as well as the effects of market-control upon practices. The chapter ends with a discussion of some pointers for further analysis of the relations between practices and market-control.

The concept of practice offers a novel approach for studying the effects of contemporary market-controls upon work activity. The decision to use the concept of practice instead of the orthodox language and concepts provided by the professions literature is justified for the following reasons. The concept of practice allows more scope than the professions literature to study work activity at the individual level of analysis. The findings of this study are based on analysing individual doctors, scientists and engineers experiences of working under conditions of market-control. The concept of practice offers possibilities for more comparative studies of work. Whilst the work referred to in this chapter is that of 'professionalised occupations' and 'professionals', the concept of practice is not restricted to professionalised occupations. Most important, through the related concepts of internal goods, external goods and standards of excellence the authors have been able to interpret and make sense of the work experiences of doctors, engineers and scientists working in market conditions. By doing so, conclusions have been formed about the effects of contemporary market-control upon different kinds of organizations and different kinds of work.

Supportive of Macintyre (1990) and Keat (1991), the evidence shows that practices are vulnerable to market-control. Some doctors, scientists and engineers experiences suggest that internal goods and practice standards of excellence can be undermined by reduced funding for long-term medical and scientific research. Also, meeting the demands of clients may restrict opportunities for individual learning, encourage the application of minimum quality standards, as well as discourage collegiate behaviour and open communication amongst practice colleagues.

Conversely, the evidence indicates that market forces can also enhance practice standards of excellence and offer different opportunities for practitioners to realise internal goods. Seen in a more positive light, client relations can allow practitioners opportunities to exhibit, test, and enhance their knowledge and skill. Client relations can allow practitioners to realise internal goods through new experiences, for example, many scientists and engineers welcomed the 'thrill' resulting from the direct application of their expertise to clients' problems. Most importantly perhaps, many doctors, scientists and engineers recognised that they can bring to bear upon their work the benefits of an interactive relationship with informed, knowledgeable clients. This mixed response suggests that the implications for practices of market-control are not so one dimensional as existing practice literature argues (Macintyre, 1990; Keat, 1991). The two-way direction of the arrows on figure one help to illustrate this point.

This more complex understanding of the relationship between markets and practices suggests a new set of questions for research, for example, under what conditions are practices vulnerable? under what conditions are practices enhanced? These questions would begin to direct attention to deeper complexities which inform the relationships between practices, organizations and markets. This approach may further explain practitioners varying individual and collective responses to market-control. An intellectual challenge for the future is to identify contingencies in the complex set of relationships between practitioners, organizations and markets which create effects that may undermine or enhance practices. The evidence in this chapter suggests that these contingencies involve all three points in the triangular relationship between markets, organizations and practitioners. Implicit in the evidence presented by this chapter is the argument that the effect of market control on practices depends on the character of the market which practitioners are exposed to, organizations' approach to managing practitioners, and practitioners' own work orientation, expectations and sources of fulfilment in work. For example, the internal market of the NHS (Ferlie et al. 1993) presents health-care practitioners with different pressures to those presented to scientists and engineers whose laboratories compete in unregulated, international markets. Equally, organisations can take very different approaches to managing the market and may mediate market pressures upon practitioners (Whittington, et al. 1994). Finally, practitioners possess a skill and expertise that can create highly mutual relationships with clients. Also, practitioners vary in their expectations of work and find alternative sources of satisfaction in work. Individuals' different work orientations may lead to different perceptions of client demands and whether meeting these demands constitutes a threat to the realisation of internal goods and practice ideals.

Notes

We are grateful for comments received about earlier versions of this chapter from Professors Armand Hatchuel, Andrew Pettigrew, and Tony Watson. Also for those received at the 11th EGOS Colloquium, 1993, and 'Professions and Management in Britain conference', University of Stirling, 1993.

This research was funded by the Economic and Social Research Council (ESRC).

References

Abercrombie, N. (1991), 'The privilege of the producer', in R. Keat and N. Abercrombie (eds), *Enterprise culture*, London, Routledge.

Abbott, A. (1988), *The system of professions*, Chicago, University of Chicago Press.

Bailyn, L. (1985), 'Autonomy in the industrial R & D lab', *Human Resource Management*, 24, pp. 129-146.

Berger, P. L. and Luckmann, T. (1967), *The social construction of reality*, Anchor, New York.

Bloor, G. and Dawson, P. (1994), 'Understanding Professional Culture in the Organisational Context' *Organization Studies* 15/2,pp. 275-295.

Crompton, R. (1990), 'Professions in the current context', *Work, Employment & Society*, Special Issue, May, pp. 147-166.

Dawson, S., Mole, V., Winstaley, D. and Sherval, J. (1992), 'Management competition and professional practice: medicine and the market place'. Paper given at the 'Knowledge workers in contemporary organizations' Conference, University of Lancaster', 1992.

Department of Health (1989), *Working for Patients*, HMSO, London.

Drazin, R. (1990), 'Professionals and innovation: structural-functional versus radical-structural perspectives', *Journal of Management Studies*, 23, 3, pp. 245-263.

Du Gay, P. and Salaman, G. (1992), 'The cult(ure) of the customer', *Journal of Management Studies*, 29, 5, pp. 615-633.

Elliot, P. (1973), 'Professional ideology and social situation', *Sociological Review*, 21.

Ferlie, E., Cairncross, L. and Pettigrew, A. (1993), 'Introducing market like mechanisms in the public sector: the case of the national health service', in L. Zan, S. Zambon, and A. Pettigrew (eds) *Perspectives on Strategic Change*, Kluwer.

Halal, W., Geranmayeh, A. and Pourdehnad, J. (1993), *Internal markets* New York, Wiley.

Harrison, S. (1988), *Managing the national health service: shifting the frontier?*. London, Chapman & Hall.

Keat, R. (1991), 'Consumer sovereignty and the integrity of practices', in Keat, R. and Abercrombie, N. (eds), *Enterprise Culture*, London, Routledge.

Lane, R. E. (1991), *The Market Experience*, Cambridge, Cambridge University Press.

Larson, M. S. (1977), *The Rise of Professionalism: A Sociological Analysis*, London, University Of California Press.

Lebas, M. and Weigenstein, J. (1986), 'Management control: the roles of rules, markets and culture', *Journal of Management Studies*, 259-272.

MacIntyre, A. (1990), *After virtue: a study in moral theory*, London, Duckworth.

Ouchi, W. (1980), 'Markets, bureaucracies and clans', *Administrative Science Quarterly*, March, Vol 25, (1) pp. 129-141.

Raelin, J. (1985), The basis for professionals resistance to managerial control, *Human Resource Management*, 24, pp. 129-146.

Reed, M. (1992), *The Sociology of Organisations*, London, Harvester-Wheatsheaf.

Reed, M. (1989), *The Sociology of Management*, London, Harvester-Wheatsheaf.

Reed, M. (1985), *Redirections in Organisational Analysis*, London, Tavistock.

Ritti, R. R. (1971), *The Engineer in the Industrial Corporation*, London, Columbia University Press.

Savage M., Dickens P., Felding T. (1988), 'Some social and political implications of the contemporary fragmentation of the 'service class' in Britain'. *International Journal of Urban and Regional Research*, 12, 3, pp. 455-475.

Scrivens, E. (1991), 'Is there a role for marketing in the public sector'? *Public Money and Management*, 11, 2, pp. 17-25.

Smith, C (1989), 'Technical workers: a class and organizational analysis, in *Organization Theory and Class Analysis*, S. Clegg (ed) New York, De Gruyter.

Sveiby, K. E. and Lloyd, T. (1987), *Managing knowhow*, London, Bloomsbury.

Torrington, D. and McKay, L. (1986), 'Will consultants take over the personnel function?'. *Personnel Management*, February, 34-27.

Watson, T. (1982), 'Group ideologies and organisational change'. *Journal of Management Studies*, 19:3, pp. 259-275.

Watson, T. (1987), *Sociology Work and Industry*, RKP, London.

Whittington, R., McNulty, T., Whipp, R. (1994), 'Market-driven change in professional services: problems and processes', *Journal of Management Studies*, Vol 31, No 6, pp. 829-844.

Whittington, R. (1992), 'Changing control strategies in industrial r & d', *R & D Management*, 21, 1, pp. 43-53.

Williamson, O.E. (1975), *Markets and hierarchies*, New York, Free Press.

Yorke, D. (1990), 'Developing an interactive approach to the marketing of professional services', in *Understanding Business Markets* D. Ford, (Eds). London, Academic Press.

Part III

DIFFERENTIATION

6 The crucial role of professional status in promoting change: the development of services for HIV/AIDS

Chris Bennett

Introduction

Although much of the management literature is focused on change, the role of professional groups in promoting change tends to be underplayed, as witness their omission from the subject indexes of some of the most influential management books of recent years (Peters and Waterman, 1982; Kanter, 1984; Pettigrew, 1987). This may well suggest that, despite the trend first commented on by Wilensky (1964) towards the 'professionalisation of everyone', it is in fact mainly the traditional professions which are thought of as such, and these, of course, are not in general visibly prominent (although many managers may originally have held professional qualifications) within the large corporations of private industry.

Thus, in order to consider the particular influence of the professional ethos on organizational change, it is necessary to look at organizations where professionals have a distinctive and powerful role in their own right, the prime examples of which are to be found in personal service organizations (Mintzberg, 1989). The focal organization of this paper, the health service, is seen by many as having always been dominated by what Strong and Robinson (1990) term the 'enormous power' of the medical profession which they see as having 'moulded every health care system in the Western industrialised world', so examination and analysis of the mechanisms by which doctors affect the process of change may well have more general application.

This paper looks at the influence of the medical profession on the development of services for a completely new and unexpected health issue, HIV/AIDS, which was first identified only just over a decade ago in a handful of patients in America. Since then, more than 600,000 cases of AIDS world-wide have been reported and many thousands of millions are being spent on prevention, treatment and care.

Although the wider implications of HIV/AIDS are not discussed in any detail in this paper, it is important to note here that the subjective impact of the epidemic has had a profound effect (Rosenburg, 1989), on individuals, organizations and society in general. HIV/AIDS has marked a return to the 'epidemic' among first world health care systems that had thought that epidemics which were not readily amenable to medical intervention and limitation were part of a past experienced by most only through hearsay and historical accounts of horrific events. In addition, many people from all walks of life found it difficult to come to terms with the association of the epidemic with long standing sexual taboos, and 'deviant' behaviours. Strong (1990) argues that 'epidemic psychology', a melange of fear, explanation/moralisation and calls for action, can 'infect' almost everyone in society: thus, in the context of this paper, it should be remembered that doctors, beneath their professional personas, are also individuals with the same capacities for experiencing fear and moral indignation and having the same propensities for unconsidered 'knee jerk' reactions as everyone else.

The history of the organizational response to HIV/AIDS in the UK can be usefully analysed as having three 'stages': a pre-legitimation stage (roughly 1981-86); a legitimation stage (1986-87) and a post legitimation stage (1987 onwards). During each of these stages an important role has been played by high status medical professionals: first in sensing the issue and mobilising an early response (stage one), secondly in acting as a focus for legitimating structures, policies an strategies (stage two) and, more recently (stage three), in either helping to sustain interest and activity in an issue which no longer grabs the headlines, or in some instances acting in a manner which may tend to inhibit further service development.

This chapter considers these different roles taken by key medical professionals at various times during the course of the epidemic so far, and seeks to show how their activities played a crucial part in the process of achieving recognition and resources for the issue during the early years of the epidemic, and in shaping the character of the services that have evolved. It argues that the success of these medical 'product champions' (Stocking, 1985) was in great part due to the archetypical characteristics of professionals, such as status, autonomy and collegiality, allied to characteristics of entrepreneurs such as single-minded drive and enthusiasm.

An interesting aspect of the medical response to the HIV/AIDS issue concerns the development of expertise in a field in which there were initially no 'experts'. Its claim to an exclusive knowledge base is, of course, an essential feature of professionalism, and the paper demonstrates the various processes by which the requisite expertise was acquired by medical professionals. In part (and probably uniquely) this happened through collaboration with patients themselves, and with voluntary sector social movement organizations. This led to the development of close working relationships and ultimately in a number of instances to the legitimtion of such relationships through the employment of people from the voluntary sector as counsellors and coordinators of services.

The chapter also discusses the proposition that this group, who may be seen as comprising a new body of HIV/AIDS professionals, initially gained much status from their close association with, and sponsorship by high status medical professionals, and that, partly as a result, they had a major impact on service development. However, such posts, rare at first, were later encouraged by government funding policy, and the establishment of HIV/AIDS posts in health authorities where there had to date been little service development meant that high status support from medical consultants was sometimes lacking. In such cases, it is argued, coordinators were frequently unable to have the same degree of impact on the change process.

Methodological approach

The empirical foundation for this paper is data on the development of services for HIV/AIDS in England, Scotland and Wales collected over the last seven years by researchers at the Centre for Corporate Strategy and Change (CCSC), University of Warwick. It comprises major case studies of the responses of seven district health authorities (two in London, four in English provincial cities, and one in Scotland) to the need to develop services for HIV/AIDS, two smaller studies (in other English cities) focusing on particular aspects of that response, and data collected during a review of HIV/AIDS services across Wales on behalf of the Welsh office.

The theoretical orientation underpinning the research was that of contextualism, the analysis of organizational change in terms of the context and process, as well as its content. Originally proposed by Pepper (1942), the contextualist approach to longitudinal field research on change has been a feature of the work of the CCSC since its establishment in 1985 and has been described in a number of publications, most recently Pettigrew (1990). The contextualist approach recognises and can deal with change as an essentially messy and untidy process, where there are often high levels of uncertainty about progress and outcome. The aim of the data collection is to allow an analysis of the process which is not purely chronological but will go beyond this to identify patterns in the process as they develop over time, to address the 'how' and 'why' as well as the 'what' of service change.

A good example of the contextualist approach as applied to healthcare organizations is that described in Pettigrew, Ferlie and McKee (1992). This work on change issues in the NHS initiated the stream of research on the development of services for HIV/AIDS on which this chapter is based. Data collected using this approach are longitudinal and qualitative, allowing for both retrospective and real time analysis, and most frequently using the case study as a research strategy because this form of empirical enquiry has specific advantages when explanations are sought concerning contemporary events over which the investigator has little or no control. Although time and resource constraints mean an inevitable trade-off between sample size and depth of analysis, and at their best case studies can capture the richness of context and process in a way that is distinctively different, and may for some purposes be more useful than data collected using more quantitative methods and larger samples (Yin, 1989). In fact Miller and Friesen (1982) have argued that if the material is valuable, even a single case study can sometimes be adequate. Certainly, in this instance, given the complexity of both the HIV/AIDS issue and the host organizations, it is argued that superficial analyses could have at best provided only limited information and at worst might have been profoundly misleading.

Professionalism and organizational change: the case of HIV/AIDS

In this, the main section of the chapter, the accumulated data on the development of services for HIV/AIDS is utilised to highlight the important roles played by members of the medical profession in influencing change[1]. It begins by setting the scene through a consideration of some general characteristics of medical professionals, and something of the historical background of the key medical specialties which became involved in the response to HIV/AIDS. Following this each of the three 'stages' of the epidemic identified earlier is considered, linking the developing chronological progression of events to the activities of key individuals and interest groups.

However, it is also important to be aware throughout that, particularly during the early years, many of those who saw the importance of HIV and were prepared to respond were lone voices, even within their own specialties. There were many doubters, and still are, who have represented a countervailing influence, and the use of professional status in preventing and stonewalling change is discussed in the final section.

Medical professionals

Professionals have been described as elite groups of powerful individuals (Mills, 1956) characterised by defining attributes such as autonomy and expertise, and holding particular shared moral norms of conduct (Wilensky, 1964), and medicine is often cited as the archetypical example of a 'profession'. Its members are seen as, first and foremost, part of a scientific culture (Mishler, 1981) and preeminent in their knowledge of the field of health and illness (Freidson, 1988). Doctors are highly regarded by a public which sees itself as dependent on the profession for the technological help required to restore and maintain optimum physical (and possibly mental) function, and trusts in the perceived ideals of professional service to deliver whatever interventions are required (Parsons, 1951).

However, not all doctors have equivalent status, and this has been important in the context of HIV/AIDS which has, as will be discussed, frequently had most impact on the traditionally less prominent specialties. While medicine is a high status professionalised occupation in its own right, it traditionally carries within it a ranking system which confers extra prestige and associated increased autonomy on some of its members. This status hierarchy is in part explicit (ie. there are different grades of doctors, from house officers to consultants); but it is in part implicit, though clearly understood by members of the profession, and is based on the different specialties or 'segments' (Bucher and Strauss, 1961) to which individual doctors become affiliated as they develop further expertise in a particular area.

In effect each segment contains a separate organizational identity, and its members become closer to one another than they are to doctors in other specialties (Freidson, 1970). Certain specialties are understood to be more important than others, so that a consultant neuro-surgeon, for instance, is considered 'higher' than a general surgeon, who in turn has higher status than an anaesthetist. In addition, teaching hospitals have a higher status than non-teaching hospitals, and a clinical post in either is generally seen to be more prestigious than a move into public health medicine or general practice. There is competition for posts in the higher status specialties.

This implicit, but well recognised, hierarchy contributes to what Bucher and Stelling (1977) identified as the major pressures for conflict which may arise between segments, which they (in contrast to other views of professions which stress their cohesiveness and collegiality), saw as sources of inter professional difference and of conflict, pursuing different objectives in different manners and only held together with some effort.

However, they do concede that there are also potential mechanisms for integration as there is continuous face to face bargaining between the factions, a search for allies and for compromise, and a norm of gentlemanly (*sic*) behaviour. There are also more pragmatic reasons for co-operation, as Kinston (1983) makes very clear, pointing out that there is a necessity to share technological resources, diagnostic services, ancillary staff and, of course, patients who are referred between specialist staff as and when required. Indeed, as Mintzberg (1989) points out, it is unnecessary and probably misleading to see the two models, political or collegial, as existing in isolation:

neither common interest nor self interest will dominate decision processes all the time; some combination is naturally to be expected. Professionals may agree on goals yet conflict over how they should be achieved; alternatively consensus can sometimes be achieved even where goals differ....
Political success sometimes requires a collegial posture - one must cloak self interest in the mantle of the common good. Likewise, collegial ends sometimes require political means.

Thus the discussion so far presents a picture of medical professionals as people with considerable individual status and autonomy, based on a general expertise in delivering medical care. These, as they develop further competence in particular aspects of medicine, become affiliated to traditional medical specialties within which and between which can be identified mechanisms of both conflict and consensus, isolationism and cooperation.

Key medical specialties affected by HIV/AIDS

The foregoing indicates that the response of medical professionals to HIV/AIDS has to be seen as developing within a specific organizational context, the medical specialty. HIV/AIDS, initially at least, had hardly any impact on some specialties, whereas its effect on others has been so great as to change them out of all recognition. Here a brief look is taken at the historical development of these key service settings, reaching back in some instances long before the beginning of this century, during which specialties developed the individual characteristics which were later to have a critical impact on their response to HIV/AIDS.

The medical specialties most closely involved with the HIV/AIDS issue to date have been, on the clinical side, genito-urinary medicine, infectious diseases, haemophilia and drugs services; and one non-clinical specialty, public health. Sometimes there were already established linkages between groupings, for others this was not the case, and individual specialties had developed from quite different traditions. However, there was one linking factor which, though clearly coincidental, was of considerable importance in terms of the response to HIV/AIDS; they could all be seen as, to some extent, 'Cinderella specialties' within the health service hierarchy. There were a number of reasons for this, embedded in the historical development of the different specialties.

Infectious diseases as a specialty had its roots in the old isolation hospitals of the 18th and 19th centuries when few effective treatments for even common infections were available, and management was focused on prevention of spread of infection. In consequence, from very early on there was a close association between infectious diseases (including sexually transmitted diseases) and public health. This association was institutionalised following the Public Health Act in 1875 when Medical Officers of Health based in Local Authority departments were given overall responsibility for the running of most hospital and clinic services. However, at the inception of the NHS in 1948 clinical specialties became the responsibility of hospital boards, marking, according to the Acheson Report (DHSS, 1988), the beginning of 'a process of debilitation of the specialty of public health medicine'.

However, this was not the only reason for the decline of public health. Infectious diseases were themselves in decline following the advent of antibiotics and vaccines. Where previously whole wards had been set aside for the treatment of one specific illness, such as syphilis, diphtheria or poliomyelitis; by the 1960s many hospitals had only one ward set aside for dealing with infectious cases, and treatment and cure was so simple and swift in most instances that a somewhat cavalier attitude had developed generally towards preventing spread of infection. This attitude was typified by the stance which had begun to be taken by many to sexually transmitted diseases, that they were simply a readily curable health hazard of a permissive approach to casual sex (Shilts, 1987). The once important specialities of both infectious diseases and genito-urinary medicine, thus became marginalised in comparison with other acute sector specialties, such as surgery or general medicine, which had been boosted by the new interventions made possible by the technological advances of the post war years.

The relative marginality of the other two clinical specialties connected with HIV/AIDS was attributable to different causes. For haemophilia the reason was simple, it was, and always had been, a small specialty because haemophilia is a rare disease. Drugs services, on the other hand, had two reasons for being seen as a Cinderella specialty. First, they were a branch of psychiatry, not itself a front runner in the prestige stakes, and secondly few people enjoyed dealing with drug users who were perceived as very difficult and demanding patients.

Thus these specialties often did not (at least prior to HIV/AIDS) represent attractive career options for medical professionals, and clinical staff in these groupings were historically frequently isolated from decision making at the core of the organization (Strong and Berridge, 1990) sometimes having little faith in their own ability to affect events. In addition, in terms of generating organizational change, they often had even less experience of operating at a 'strategic level' than their contemporaries in the more glamorous specialties.

The situation in these specialties at the beginning of the 1980's would not have given much grounds for optimism about a future rise in status. Haemophilia was a small specialty and likely to remain so. During the 1970s the care of and prognosis for haemophiliacs had been transformed by the discovery of Factor VIII, a blood clotting factor which extracted from whole blood and injected prevented major bleeds and allowed patients to live a normal life. The treatment was simple and effective, and even the top specialist centres were run by very few staff.

Drugs services had moved from a permissive attitude to prescribing in the 60s to an approach based on requiring total abstinence in the 70s. Neither approach was seen as effective and the focus had moved from medical intervention to encouraging the involvement of voluntary organizations. Many psychiatric services offered no specialist input to drug users at all.

In genito-urinary medicine, despite the large increase in the incidence of sexually transmitted diseases during the 1970s facilities were desperately inadequate throughout the country. In Birmingham, for instance, England's 'second city', the GU clinic operated from a building the size of two portacabins sited underneath a concrete multi-storey car park and dealt with half of all cases seen across the whole NHS West Midlands Region. There had long been plans to upgrade facilities, but the low status specialty was not a front runner in the competition for resources.

The situation in infectious diseases was not quite so bad, as a number of departments had extended their remit to include tropical medicine which, with increasing travel to exotic locations, was becoming something of a growth industry. None the less, the specialty was not a prominent one and did not attract large resources. In addition, the influence of many departments was diminished by their location in the old fever hospitals some distance away from the new District General Hospitals.

The other specialty with a potential role in epidemics, public health medicine, had been badly demoralised by two NHS reorganizations, and some districts had no department of public health at all. The Acheson Report (DHSS, 1988) summarises the situation during that period:

> In some parts of the country community physicians seized the opportunity which was presented to them in 1974 and created vigorous departments ... In other places, some simply failed to make the transition. The outdated approach of some community physicians, coupled with confused lines of accountability within multi-district areas ... exacerbated by the paucity of resources available in some places, impeded the proper discharge of the public health function

It would have been difficult to put together another group of specialties which seemed collectively so unlikely to make a major impact on service development. Despite these initial disadvantages however, some medical professionals in these specialities have played key roles in the response to HIV/AIDS, and in the rest of this section some of the mechanisms by which they achieved this are examined.

1981-1985: Sensing and championing change, the roles played by medical professionals

The first stage of the organizational response to the HIV/AIDS issue, was characterised by individual initiatives and ad hoc development, but little in the way of formal recognition or financial support, and came to an end around 1986-87, when national policy on HIV/AIDS began to take shape, and formal structures were instituted to implement guidelines.

Given, therefore, that until that time HIV/AIDS was not officially recognised as an issue for the Health Service, the fundamental question about the process of change that is addressed in this section is 'how did activity around HIV/AIDS become legitimated?' The data suggest that one crucial influence on the development of the organizational response during this period was the activities of key medical professionals in first sensing and then championing the issue.

Sensing the issue: the role played by a 'scientific' medical culture

As Johnson and Scholes (1984) point out, the awareness of a strategic problem usually occurs at an individual level, and HIV/AIDS was no exception. Six of the case studies of the empirical database for this paper were deliberately selected because they were perceived to have made a particularly early response to the issue. All these were health authorities in large university cities containing several major acute hospitals, and with one exception they were also teaching authorities.

In such settings are traditionally found the medical specialists who are at the forefront of their professions, are involved in research programmes of their own, and take a keen interest in the latest developments in their specialties throughout the world. It was amongst this group that the first glimmerings of awareness of a new health problem began. One consultant remembered attending a conference on immunology at which early cases of what was later diagnosed as AIDS were presented, even before the first reports of cases were published in 1981, but others were aware of the issue almost as early through reading specialist journals:

> I was aware that it was going to be hitting Britain even in 81-82 because I've been an avid reader of M M W R ... so as soon as HIV came on the horizon I certainly knew about it.

Initially no one was even certain that an infective agent was involved, and it was mainly immunologists who were interested in the syndrome, but the established traditions of medical and scientific research ensured that the early cases of AIDS were recognised as 'something new' and, for this very reason, worthy of study. This early sensing of the issue, then, owed far more to the general preoccupations of the scientific establishment, what Roe (1952) in her study of the personal attributes of scientists characterised as 'the need to find out', than to prescience about the future importance of AIDS.

In 1983 it became clear that the breakdown of the immune system which characterised AIDS was caused by a sexually transmissible virus, now known as Human Immunodeficiency Virus (HIV). Now a different group of people, the virologists, became involved in the issue, and all over the world the race was on to develop a diagnostic test. This quotation from a virologist in one of the authorities we studied captures the excitement of the scientific chase generated at this time:

> from the very first finding of the HIV virus, I think we were probably the first laboratory in this country to be able to diagnose the disease. We got a copy of the sub-culture from Porton, and we started doing tests ourselves of a very simple nature which we devised ... from the very earliest days, so much so I broke all the rules in the book by using Gallo's strain, even though at that stage he was claiming to have it patented and people weren't allowed to use it. So I used it and said 'Sue me if you will'.

Patton (1990) argues that this shift in focus from immunology to virology in 'explaining' AIDS was in large part socially constructed, resulting from changing cultural metaphors about the origins of health and illness. This is an interesting meta-level perspective, but at an organizational level of analysis a simpler, if more prosaic, interpretation is suggested by our data and endorsed by Shilts' (1987) account of the development of the epidemic in America. That is, that by 1983 awareness of and interest in the HIV/AIDS issue was being generated at least as much by competition amongst scientists for the kudos involved in being credited with a new discovery, as by 'pure' scientific curiosity.

111

The doctor quoted in the above example had little direct involvement with patients, for others, however, there was less of a distinction between research and clinical concerns. Another aspect of the medical scientific culture in our authorities that tended to facilitate early awareness of the issue was that the application of expertise in one area sometimes led to early recognition of a problem in another.

Thus in 1982 one consultant had sought and obtained research funding to investigate the possibility of immune suppression in haemophiliacs. When the first diagnostic tests for HIV were being developed he had sequential serum samples already available, allowing early identification of HIV infection among his patients. Similarly, testing the samples of blood serum stored by doctors with a scientific research interest in the spread of Hepatitis B amongst drug users (Peutherer et al., 1985; Robertson et al., 1986) led to the early realisation that Lothian had a very large incidence of HIV infection amongst this group of patients.

Clinical 'product champions'

Arguably, this early interest in HIV/AIDS owed more to the general freedom of high status medical scientists to indulge their scientific curiosity, and the excitement of competition to make new discoveries, than to commitment to the specific issue itself. However, there were others who, for reasons varying from the personal to the altruistic, found in HIV/AIDS a new and totally absorbing interest and mission.

The 'product champion' has been found to be an important element of the innovation process in both industrial (Rothwell, 1976) and health care settings (Stocking, 1985). A product champion (Burgelman and Sayles, 1986) is seen as being able to work effectively in a non programmed environment. HIV/AIDS was certainly uncharted territory and in all the major case study districts medical 'product champions', many of them clinical consultants in the key specialties, emerged to drive forward proposals for development.

What is interesting here is that although, as noted earlier, these were low status specialties, the individual characteristics of the champions enabled them to overcome this disadvantage and exert enormous influence on their organizations and at national level, long before the issue was officially recognised by government.

What were these characteristics, which set the champions apart from other colleagues in the same specialties who, despite access to the same information, did not respond, and indeed often pooh-poohed the very idea of HIV/AIDS having any relevance to their future practice? Though they were very different as individuals, they all had in common a belief in the crucial importance of HIV/AIDS, an enthusiasm for promoting greater awareness and interest in the issue, and a broad view of its relevance outside the narrow confines of medical practice.

The early clinical product champions also showed a most unusual degree of eclecticism, given the traditional reluctance of professionals to share their expertise with others. In part, this reflected the pervading lack of knowledge about the disease during the first few years. There *were* no experts and while scientists were urgently seeking to establish the basic facts about the syndrome, clinicians were faced with needing to treat patients with AIDS and having to discover by trial and error the cocktails of drugs best suited to unusual infections. Changes in knowledge about AIDS and how to treat it were so rapid that patients were sometimes as well informed as their doctors and the old 'doctor knows best' approach proved difficult to sustain:

> most major discoveries are now not published, or they are subsequently, but they're not published in the medical journals, they're published in newspapers. That puts us at a big disadvantage ... Whereas you can read the *BMJ* and the *New England Journal of Medicine* every week, at least know what's in it and look for things like that. You can't read all the papers every day and the magazines and the women's magazines carry all this as well. So it becomes almost impossible to maintain the feeling normally that you have, that you actually know more than the patients, when sometimes you actually don't.

This assault on the knowledge base of medical professionals was increased by the close involvement in the issue of the gay community, from amongst whom most of the first patients came. They were well organised and had their own information networks and quickly came to exert a significant influence on policy and practice at both local and national level with their insistence on addressing issues of confidentiality and patient rights. Clinicians committed to delivering a service began to accept the need for change, and norms of good practice began to develop through an interaction of staff and patients, providing a vector for new ideologies of health care which challenged conventional models. Ideas about promoting a patient centred approach were not new in themselves. Movements towards community care and hospice provision, and rising interest in'alternative' therapies, have been symptomatic of changing attitudes towards health care in recent years. Nevertheless, established service delivery systems can be difficult to change. HIV/AIDS had no traditions, nor did it fit neatly into any one specialty, so services could be tailored to the perceived needs of patients.

Responding to patient pressure in this way should not be seen, however, as a total transfer of professional power to other groups. This was essentially a process of high status people 'giving away' power in one direction, patient centred services, in order to keep it in another by remaining the focus of service provision, and has been a key characteristic of the development of HIV/AIDS services.

Another aspect of the eclecticism of the early product champions was demonstrated in the formation of early ad hoc working groups on HIV/AIDS. These were notable for the inclusion of different medical specialties and local authority and voluntary sector representatives, and a great contrast to the usual medically dominated structure of advisory groups on clinical issues. In part their multidisciplinary character was undoubtedly due to the lack of widespread interest in HIV/AIDS within the specialties at that time and the determination of the voluntary sector lobby to be included, but there was also evident a vision amongst key clinicians of an appropriate future development for services.

This sense of vision, so characteristic of entrepreneurs of all kinds as they seek to attain, not only change, but a new concept (Mintzberg, 1989) resulted in a determination to develop the kinds of services the champions felt were needed, regardless of even the most protracted opposition, and some were prepared to use every means at their disposal to manipulate the situation:

> I recognised early on that the only way we'd get [funders] to move was to embarrass them, and ... we got onto the newspapers and the box and turned the temperature up and got them to respond.

This suggests that one method used by key medical professionals in order to achieve change was that of crisis construction. As Pettigrew (1983) noted, there are:

> Real and constructed crises, the latter are brought about for the express purpose of facilitating change, and involve mobilising elements of a context, extracting and shaping from the context a justification and a language for making things happen.

There were, of course, plenty of real crises occurring during the early years of HIV/AIDS, ranging from media fuelled outbreaks of fear and anxiety amongst staff in London hospitals with early clinical cases, to the sudden revelation of large numbers of infected drug users in Lothian. However, key medical professionals quickly became seen as 'experts' (as Handy (1976) points out, anyone is an expert who knows more than anyone else around), and developed skill in presenting the very limited information available in a way calculated to create a perception of the need for change. One respondent recalled an argument with a government minister on television in 1983 or 1984:

> Now at that time about fourteen or fifteen had been diagnosed or had died with AIDS, and he was saying, 'well, how many corpses do you need, do you need twenty, a hundred, two hundred, when is it enough?', you can see what is happening in the States.

In another instance, a medical product champion used the discovery that many haemophiliac patients had been infected through receiving contaminated Factor 8 to 'construct' a local crisis around HIV/AIDS:

> Because of the way that the haemophiliacs had been infected our figures looked worse than they really were....We had an extra hundred infected people in the stats that were part of a different epidemic that had peaked, because 60 per cent of the haemophiliacs had been infected and not any more of them...It made it look as if we had more...and assuming doubling times and all that you get to

horrendous numbers quite quickly. So, in other words, we had anxiety levels out of all proportion to the numbers.

It was not always necessary to have a crisis to stimulate action, and in a few of the localities studied no local crisis ever emerged. Another technique used by the early champions of HIV/AIDS was to gather around them coalitions of other important people, particularly other medical professionals to help to further their cause. In one district, the original product champion, a consultant in genito-urinary medicine, was particularly fortunate in recruiting another comrade at arms, a community medicine specialist, at an early stage.

The energy and enthusiasm of the two together proved irresistible, and without any noticeable crisis, either real or constructed, occurring, the district forged ahead, making alliances with the city council and the voluntary sector on the way. The style of the relationships formed in this district was described by a respondent as reflecting a 'tradition of genteel behaviour' which fostered collaboration and prevented outright confrontation about differences of opinion:

> there is this ethos of the kind of 'we will behave in a certain way, won't we?' ... and the key players have that ethos. I think in a way that held things.

In another district, collaboration was sometimes brought about by the use of somewhat Machiavellian tactics, and aimed not just at gaining cooperation but at consolidating the power-base of the key actor. The following account describes the method used to call a meeting of people from different organizations to develop a joint strategy for HIV/AIDS. The convener, the local product champion, asked each nominee to forward information on the actions they had already taken on the issue, although he was by no means certain that everyone he was inviting was currently active in the field:

> ... they now had a problem, nobody was going to turn up at this meeting saying, 'We haven't done anything..' So that got an enormous flurry of activity going. Boom! Suddenly everyone was in action ... So they all turned up having done something ... it was then no longer possible to defend inaction, because there was a forum in which you had to turn up and defend it.

By taking the initiative in this way, and by offering himself to chair and his organization to service the resulting structure, the product champion ensured that he maintained and strengthened his position as the key figure on HIV/AIDS in the area.

What has been the pay off for the investment of all this energy on service change? Becoming an AIDS 'product champion' could have far reaching consequences, transforming the pace of work and long term careers, for better or for worse. The glare of publicity could have negative as well as positive consequences if a perception grew of the product champion as only a 'media doctor.' Some innovators were in essence 'climbers' (Downs, 1967). HIV/AIDS, a high profile issue, with no organizational history behind it, and money available for new development, was custom-made for those at the beginning of their careers who were hoping to make their mark early:

> at that time it suddenly became a big thing, and (people) then realised it was a good thing to be in infectious diseases as this was a disease that was going somewhere..

Although most champions were clearly committed to an altruistic vision ocombating the epidemic, it is inescapable that their motives for involvement were not unmixed with personal advancement. Many of those scorned by their contemporaries for their early obsession with HIV/AIDS - 'he's on his hobby horse again' - have more recently seen their hunches justified by invitations to sit on national committees as experts, international recognition and offers of prestigious new appointments. In addition, they have in many cases seen their specialties expanded and transformed by new capital and revenue money.

The picture of the product champion that emerges from the data, then, is not as homogeneous as one might have thought. They differed in both individual character and styles of management. Some were skilled at diplomacy and coalition building, while others found the best way to overcome opposition was to ignore it, or to use personal clout to railroad people into co-operating, and there were even some whose ability to alienate the very people they wished to influence was legendary.

What they all had, however, was a quality that Peters and Waterman (1982) identified as a key attribute of the champion, the ability to take responsibility for converting ideas into action. The champions were the doers. They set up the *ad hoc* committees, they went ahead with getting people together and telling them about AIDS, they set up services on shoestrings by bending existing services to fit (often without waiting for permission), and they were prepared to work longer and harder than almost anyone else to achieve their goals.

1985-1987: A legitimating role for medical professionals, the creation of a structural response

Those perceived to have the power to heal have always held individually influential positions in their societies, but in this century doctors have increasingly practiced within institutional frameworks (for a review of this historical development see Starr, 1982, or Freidson, 1970). Some writers (such as Esland, 1980) have seen this increasing dependence on structure as necessitating a diminution of the power and autonomy of the medical profession, but others, while acknowledging some loss of autonomy, have seen doctors as having been able to make political use of that structure to negotiate their status with government so that they can act largely unhampered by managerial controls (Freddi, 1989).

In order to maintain this degree of privilege and in order to legitimate and protect their own professional structures and operational standards doctors have had to become closely involved in the political process. Hence, since the beginning of the welfare state and the institution of the NHS, the medical profession, and in particular representatives of those who work in the field of public health have worked closely with and in government departments. There may have been some loss of autonomy, but the opportunity to influence and often determine government policy on health care has probably been seen as compensatory, at least by those privileged to walk in the corridors of power.

A key role for public health

Thus when the issue of AIDS first arose, and government became aware of a potential health crisis to which it must respond, it was to this group of public health physicians that ministers and government officials turned for guidance, and the Chief Medical Officer, Sir Donald Acheson, received much praise for his handling of the issue. The approach taken is well illustrated by the heading to an article by Polly Toynbee in the Guardian in March 1987:

> No moralising, no politics - just a no-nonsense, medically based campaign. This was how Sir Donald Acheson tackled the Cabinet.

Hence, as Fox et al., (1989) put it, the social construction of the epidemic at government level as a professional issue meant that it was defined as mainly a problem for the experts and could be seen as 'an unseemly subject for partisan debate'.

Thus, by 1986, the role of professional public health doctors at government level in the response to the epidemic was already seen as legitimate and powerful. It was now the turn of public health physicians at health authority level to take centre stage, as a Department of Health Circular (DHSS, 1986) was issued directing 'Standing action groups' on AIDS to be formally constituted in every district:

> accountable to the health authority through a nominated community physician, to be responsible for co-ordinating relevant local services and spearheading prevention.

The directive was, in essence, a public health physicians charter, signalling that they were expected to take over the managerial reins, if that were not already the case. Although HIV/AIDS was clearly above everything a public health issue, and arguably concerned prevention far more than treatment and care, relatively few public health physicians had taken an early lead. This meant that during the early years, decisions about service development for HIV/AIDS had tended to be taken on the hoof by the medical product champions, (mostly clinicians), or with the minimum of bureaucratic procedure through their ad hoc committees.

So the formation of the action committees imposed a clear framework and lines of accountability on an issue that was threatening to develop in a very uncoordinated way in response to the interests of key movers in the districts. This had three main effects; it re-emphasised HIV/AIDS as a medical issue; it gave a new impetus to prevention; and it created a bureaucratic buffer between clinicians championing the cause and general management, both at district and regional level.

The last of these had the most immediate effect. Until then, key physicians had been able to use their influence to gain support for HIV/AIDS from whoever was prepared to listen, an approach hallowed by tradition amongst consultants:

> Our approach over the years was always to identify what we thought we should be doing and then go along the road and bang on the door and reach the table and say 'this is what we need ... stuff you and the problems you have got, we are the ones at ground level and we know what we want.'

Much of the early service development for HIV/AIDS had come about by such means. Unit general managers had been cornered and persuaded to fund expansion of departments, research grants had been used to pump prime service delivery, representatives of voluntary bodies had been used by clinicians to lobby ministers for funds for hospital services, and (usually as a last resort) local needs had been hyped to the media. Now public health physicians were to act as the gatekeepers for requests, and had overall responsibility for balancing the different demands.

For all the community medicine specialists in the sample of early responding health authorities from which this data is taken, this was the turning point, the moment from which they began to play a most important, possibly the most important part in service development for HIV/AIDS. It was now possible, in theory at least, to put a gentle brake on over-enthusiastic suggestions for service development in the acute sector (one district was making plans for a 50 bedded custom-built unit at a notional cost of £1-3 million) and to start to consider the needs for prevention treatment and care at a more strategic level.

Thus HIV/AIDS, having boosted the careers of some clinicians and the prestige of some under-rated specialties now provided a new key managerial role and opportunities for advancement for public health.

1987-199?: Holding the ring, the role played by medical professionals in sustaining interest and commitment

The mid to late 1980s was a period of great enthusiasm and high activity. HIV/AIDS had been established as a high status issue in its own right; government departments and committees were focusing on it; those who had been early in the field were now in demand as experts; and a number of previously neglected specialties were enjoying a considerable renaissance. Central funding was now instituted, and with ear-marked allocations rising rapidly from £8.1 million in 1985 to £137.3 million in 1990-91, arguing the need for service development became less difficult, particularly where authorities had already established themselves as leaders in the field.   On the other hand, the need to manage the issue became more apparent. It did not always prove easy to take a strategic view of service development. First, the shape of the epidemic itself was rapidly changing, with increasing anxieties about heterosexual spread. Then the issue proposed many intra and inter organizational boundaries and the people involved all had their own particular interests and perspectives and sometimes very different ideologies as well. A problem with individual change agents is that they frequently expect to achieve their ends through familiar means, and within their own span of control. The early activities of product champions had tended to foster service infrastructures which, while often very innovative, were based on specific acute sector departments. Managing HIV/AIDS sometimes involved putting a brake on development in one area in order to respond to changing circumstances and needs elsewhere, sometimes occasioning controversy.

Another task for managers, with the HIV/AIDS ring-fenced allocation representing just about the only growth area in the health service, was trying to determine what were, or were not, appropriate calls on the budget. Improved standards for control of cross-infection were a high priority, but should the money really come from the HIV/AIDS allocation, or from base budgets? How did one deal tactfully with opportunistic requests to fund items with somewhat tenuous connections with HIV?

It was here that status struggles became evident. As mentioned earlier, the recognition of HIV/AIDS as an important issue did not just raise anxiety levels amongst the general public, but gave rise to all sorts of concerns amongst members of the medical profession, and in particular surgeons, about the possibility of transmission of infection. Public health consultants, even in a managerial role, often found it very hard to withstand pressure from traditionally elite specialties demanding new equipment, or extra money to fund what many people saw as excessively elaborate precautions when operating. One public health respondent, despite being a most influential figure in his own right, admitted to sometimes feeling 'rather like putty in the hands of a powerful surgical group'.

The new agents of change, HIV professionals

Another feature of this boom period in HIV service development was a realisation that not only dedicated structures, but dedicated posts neede to be created. In districts that had been early in responding to the issue, this had been clear for some time. The multiplicity of service developments were far outstripping the management capability of even the most dedicated clinical product champions, and public health physicians had other responsibilities besides HIV/AIDS. Those applying for the early posts were frequently young, bright, enthusiastic and had activist leanings, Many had also already been involved with voluntary initiatives for HIV/AIDS and had developed relationships with key medical professionals involved with service delivery.

Both individually and collectively, the new generation of HIV/AIDS workers made a big impact on the statutory organizations. Since by all ordinary standards, hierarchical status, span of control, even possession of expertise, they should have had little influence, we need to ask why this was so. One key factor was that they had powerful allies, being appointed, for the most part, by important product champions who both protected and gave them autonomy to develop their roles. Then, their job titles frequently included words like 'co-ordinator', 'facilitator' or 'liaison', which implicitly invested them with the power to cross inter and intra sectoral boundaries and to mediate between the various interest groups.

Another important attribute was that they often did not belong to any particular professional group, or if they did, were not using their professional skills in traditional ways, so others were neither intimidated by their superior status, nor dismissive of them as inferior. Also they were frequently birds of passage, committed to the task, but not to the institution, and therefore with little to lose by confronting difficult and controversial issues. Finally, and perhaps most importantly, they were able to give their full time and attention to the task, which few of the early advocates of the cause had been able to do.

The way in which key medical professionals were able, in effect to 'lend' status to others outside the profession is interesting, since although this process has been described in terms of patronage within the medical fraternity (Hall, 1949; Freidson, 1970), there has been little discussion of the possibility of this being effective across disciplinary boundaries. However, the proposition that powerful sponsorship seems to have been an important factor in the influence wielded by the early HIV professionals is further evidenced by current circumstances.

Improvements in the financial situation and government support for coordinator posts focusing particularly on aspects of prevention and health education have led to appointments being made in most health authorities, but many post holders are now working in districts where there are still no powerful medical champions for the issue. Now individual workers with no status of their own and lacking powerful sponsors are tending to find they are much less influential at management level, and many are becoming progressively disenchanted with their ability to affect service development.

HIV drops down the agenda. can professional status help?

The current plight of HIV co-ordinators mirrors a more general drop in interest which, perversely, coincided with the arrival in 1989, of the really large amounts of central funding for HIV/AIDS which had long been requested by those involved in service development. By this time, however, there were indications that cases of AIDS were not increasing as fast as had been predicted (PHLS, 1990) and this fuelled suspicion that some had been 'crying wolf' in order to boost their specialties. In addition, management attention had been diverted to implementation of the new NHS reforms.

Thus, far from the new money heralding a new period of service expansion, those involved in HIV/AIDS found its status (and to some degree their own) dropping, and rapidly became involved in fighting a rearguard action to avoid some of the new allocation being vired to other more prestigious specialties currently under financial pressure. The situation was saved, but only by government intervention through the National Audit Office (NAO, 1991), with district general managers being reminded that HIV/AIDS money was ringfenced and could not be used for other purposes. The message is plain, HIV/AIDS had a special status of its own, has lost it, and seems unlikely to regain it to any great extent in the foreseeable future, despite the assertion in *The Health of the Nation* (1991) that HIV/AIDS is 'the greatest new threat to public health this century'.

This is interesting in the context of the theme of this paper, which has suggested that it was the status (and the autonomy that this ensured) inherent in the positions of key medical actors which was to a great extent responsible for the HIV/AIDS issue's rise to prominence during the early years. It seems that, once prominence had been achieved, those professionals and their once backwater specialties gained further status by association with what they had helped to create. The question which has yet to be answered is whether, as the issue itself declines in perceived importance, those associated with it will lose all they have gained, or whether the investment which has been made in their specialties will have raised their general status sufficiently to ensure, for example, that genito-urinary medicine will continue to attract young career orientated doctors, rather than simply those who have failed to get positions elsewhere.

What role can the key medical professionals now play in promoting change in HIV/AIDS? Do they indeed still wish to do so? The problem with championing a cause is in maintaining the momentum over long periods. Ferlie (1993) has suggested that there may be a search for second generation leadership because of burn out, and Street (1993) points to a possible playing out of Downs' (1967) 'issue attention cycle'. It may be that the role of the medical professionals is now in providing the needed continuity that their privileged position in tenured posts provides, irrespective of their internal status within their profession; and in being prepared, as they were when HIV/AIDS arose as a brand new health issue, to recognise and respond to new crises as and when they may arise.

Concluding remarks

This chapter has used research on the development of services for HIV/AIDS to trace some aspects of the involvement of medical professionals in the issue from its inception to the current time.

It argues that high status professionals have played a very important role in first sensing and then championing the cause of HIV/AIDS, and that the rise in the profile of this issue, for which they were partly responsible, has led to both themselves, and their comparatively low status specialties acquiring further status as a consequence of their association with it.

It further argues that, as well as having a key role in promoting change themselves, high status professionals may also have a very important part to play in facilitating change through their sponsorship of others with lower status who are not themselves doctors. This possibility is not explicitly addressed in the literature.

In conclusion the chapter poses some questions about the role of high status professionals in stabilising and maintaining the momentum of service development.

Some of these findings are interesting and potentially important outside as well as inside the health service. It is suggested that further research on the role of professional status in promoting change in other private and public sector settings is required to see if these findings are applicable more generally.

Notes

1. It should be noted that although the involvement of medical professionals was crucial, it is not suggested that the stimulus their efforts provided was the only factor in the change process. Discussion of other motivators of change and the broader context affecting the HIV/AIDS issue can be found in Bennett and Pettigrew (1991); Bennett (1992); Ferlie and Bennett (1992) and Ferlie (1993).

References

Bennett, C. E. (1992), 'HIV/AIDS: Some Organizational and Managerial Issues' *Journal of Management in Medicine*, Vol. 6, No. 4, pp. 40-45.

Bennett, C. E. and Pettigrew, A. M. (1991), *Pioneering services for Aids: The response to HIV infection in four health authorities*, Final Report of research for Department of Health CCSC, University of Warwick, pp. 61.

Bucher, R. and Stelling, J. (1977), 'Characteristics of Professional Organizations' in Blankenship, R.L. (ed.), *Colleagues in Organisations*, London, John Wiley, pp. 121-144.

Bucher, R. and Strauss, A. (1961), 'Professions in Process', *American Journal of Sociology*, 66, 325-334.

Burgelman, R. A. and Sayles, L. R. (1986), *Inside Corporate Innovation: Strategy. Structure and Managerial Skills*, London, Collier Macmillan.

DHSS (1986), *Resource Assumptions and Planning Guidelines*, Health Circular, HC (86) 2.

DHSS (1988), *Public Health in England: The Report of the Committee of Enquiry into the Future Development of the Public Health Function*, (Cmnd. 289), London, HMSO, (1988), (The Acheson Report).

Downs, A. (1967), *Inside Bureaucracies*, Little Brown Company, Boston.

Esland, G. (1980), 'Professions and professionalism' in Esland, G. and Salamon, G (eds), *The politics of work and occupations*, Milton Keynes, Open University Press.

Ferlie, E. B. (1993), 'The Response to AIDS by British District Health Authorities' in Strong, P. and Berridge, V. (eds), *AIDS and Contemporary History*, Cambridge, Cambridge University Press.

Ferlie, E. B. and Bennett, C. E. (1992), 'Patterns of strategic change in health care: District Health Authorities respond to AIDS', *British Journal of Management*, Vol. 3, pp. 21-37.

Fox, D. M., Day, P. and Klein, R. (1989), 'The power of professionalism: policies for AIDS in Britain, Sweden, and the United States', *Daedulus*, Vol. 118, No. 2, Spring 1989.

Freddi, G. (1989), 'Problems of organizational rationality in health systems: Political controls and policy options' in Freddi, G. and Bjorkman, J.W. (1989), *Controlling medical professionals: The comparative politics of health governance*, London, Sage Publications.

Freidson, E. (1970), *Professional Dominance: the Social Structure of Medical Care*, Atherton Press, New York.

Freidson, E. (1988), *Profession of medicine: a study of the sociology of applied knowledge (with a new aforeword)*, University of Chicago Press.

Hall, O. (1949), 'Types of medical career', *American Journal of Sociology*, LV pp. 243-253.

Handy, C. (1976), *Understanding organisations*, Penguin Books Ltd., Harmondsworth.

Johnson, G. and Scholes, K. (1984), *Exploring corporate strategy*, London, Prentice-Hall International Inc.

Johnson, G. and Scholes, K. (1992), *Exploring corporate strategy*, 3rd edition, London, Prentice-Hall International Inc.

Kanter, R. M. (1984), *The change masters: Corporate entrepreneurs at work*, George Allen and Unwin.

Kinston, W. (1983), 'Hospital organization and structure and its effect on inter professional behaviour and the delivery of care' *Social Science of Medicine*, Vol. 17, No. 16, pp. 1169-1170.

Miller, D. and Friesen, P. M. (1982), 'The Longitudinal Analysis of Organizations: A Methodological Perspective', *Management Science*, 28, 9, 1,013-34.

Mills, C. W. (1956), *The power elite*, New York, OUP.

Mintzberg, H. (1989), *Mintzberg on Management*, New York, Free Press.

Mintzberg, H., Brunet, J. P. and Waters, J. (1986), 'Does planning impede strategic thinking?' *Advances in Strategic Management*, Vol. 4, JAI Press, Greenwich CT 1986, pp. 3-41.

Mishler, E. G. (1981), 'Critical perspectives on the bio-medical model' in Mishler, E. G., Singham, M. A., Hauser, S. T., Liem, R., Osherson, S. D. and Waxler, N. E. (eds), *Social contexts of health illness and patient care*, Cambridge, Cambridge University Press.

Morgan, G. (1986), *Images of organisation*, London, Sage Publications.

National Audit Office (1991), *HIV and AIDS related health services*, report by the comptroller and auditor general, London, HMSO.

Parsons, T. (1951), *The social system*, New York, The Free Press.

Patton, C. (1990), *Inventing AIDS*, London, Routledge 1990.

Pepper, S. C. (1942), *World hvpotheses*, Berkley, University of California Press.

Peters, T. and Waterman, R. H. (1982), *In search of excellence*, London, Harper and Row.

Pettigrew, A. M. (1983), 'Patterns of managerial response as organizations move from rich to poor environments', *Educational Management and Administration*, pp. 104-114.

Pettigrew, A. M. (1985a), 'Contextualist Research: A Natural Way to Link Theory and Practice', in Lawler, E. (ed.), *Doing Research that is Useful in Theory and in Practice*, San Francisco, Jossey Bass.

Pettigrew, A. M. (1985b), *The Awakening Giant*, Oxford, Basil Blackwell.

Pettigrew, A. M. (1987), *The Management of Strategic Change*, Oxford, Basil Blackwell.

Pettigrew, A. M. (1990), 'Longitudinal field research on change: Theory and practice', *Organisation Science*, Vol. 3, No. 1, 1990, pp. 267-292.

Pettigrew, A. M., Ferlie, E. B. and McKee, L. (1992), *Shaping strategic change: Making change in large organisations - the case of the NHS*', London, Sage.

Peutherer, J. F., Edmond, E., Simmonds, P., Dickson, J. D. and Bath, G. E. (1985), 'HTLV-III Antibody in Edinburgh Drug Addicts', *The Lancet*, Vol. 2, November 16 1985, pp. 1129.

Pfeffer, J. and Salancik, G. R. (1978), *The external control of organisations: A resource dependence perspective*, New York, Harper and Row.

Public Health Laboratory Service (1990), 'Acquired Immune Deficiency Syndrome in England and Wales to end 1993: projections using data to end September 1989', *Communicable Disease Report,* (the Day Report), January 1990.

Robertson, J. R., Bucknall, A. B. V., Welsby, P. D., Roberts, J. J. K., Inglis, J. M., Peutherer, J. F. and Brettle, R. P. (1986), 'Epidemic of AIDS related Virus (HTLV-III/LAV) infection amongst intravenous drug abusers', *British Medical Journal*, Vol. 292, 22 February 1986, pp. 527.

Roe, A. (1952), 'A psychologist examines sixty-four eminent scientists', *Scientific American*, Vol. 187, 1952, pp. 21-5.

Rosenberg, C. (1989), 'What is an epidemic? AIDS in historical perspective', *Daedalus*, 118, 2, pp. 1-18.

Rothwell, R. (1976), 'Intracorporate Entrepreneurs', *Management Decision*, (13), 3, pp. 142-154.

Secretary of State for Health (1991), *The Health of The Nation*, London, HMSO, 1991.

Shilts, R. (1987), *And The Band Played On*, London, Penguin.

Starr, P. (1982), 'The growth of medical authority' in Brown, P. (ed.), 1989) *Perspectives in medical sociology,* California, Wadsworth Publishing Co. Inc.

Stocking, B. (1985), *Initiative and Inertia in the NHS*, London, Nuffield Provincial Hospitals Trust.

Street, J. (1993), 'A fall in interest? British AIDS policy, 1986-1990' in Berridge, V. and Strong, P. (eds), *AIDS and contemporarv history*, Cambridge University Press.

Strong, P. (1990), 'Epidemic psychology: a model' *Sociology of Health and Illness* Vol. 12 No.3, 1990, pp. 249-259.

Strong, P. and Berridge, V. (1990), 'No one knew anything: some issues in British AIDS Policy, in Aggleton, P., Davies, P. and Hart, G. (eds), *AIDS: Individual cultural and policy dimensions,* London, Falmer Press.

Strong, P. and Robinson, J. (1990), *The NHS under new management*, Open University Press.

Wilensky, H. L. (1964), 'The professionalisation of everyone?' *American Journal of Sociology,* Vol. LXX, No. 2, September 1964.

Yin, R. K. (1989), *Case study research: design and methods,* Beverley Hills, Sage.

7 Contracts, resources and resistance to change: power and professional relations in the London teaching hospital

Ian Tilley

Introduction

This chapter forms part of a wider study of some of the organizational effects and changes to acute NHS hospitals arising from the implementation of the Government's recent health initiatives. The current policy had its main legislative expression in the *National Health Service and Community Care Act* (Department of Health, 1990). The particular focus of the Greenwich study is the inner London teaching hospital. It faces complex, concentrated change arising not only from the Government's health Reforms but also from their efforts to 'rationalize' the provision of acute services in the capital. These 'rationalization' moves are beginning to bite. They include the Tomlinson Inquiry (1992) into London's health provision; the establishment of the London Implementation Group (LIG) which is overseeing the mergers and closures of NHS hospital, medical education and research institutions until April 1995 when it hands over to the two London regional health authorities (RHAs); the LIG's specialty reviews (Butler, 1993); and the Secretary of State for Health's reaction to these reviews (DoH, 1993) and her decision on individual hospitals, including the down grading/forced merger of some of the most famous teaching hospitals in the UK. As a consequence of such moves, LIG is funding significant redundancy programmes and created a clearing house or 'dating agency' to assist nurses (and supposedly doctors too) made redundant by the restructuring find new jobs.

In the other major conurbations 'mini Tomlinsons' are in progress. So although in some ways a special case, the experience of the famous inner London teaching hospitals increasingly has a wider relevance, certainly for other big city hospitals and even beyond that.

The approach taken in the whole Greenwich study is presented in Salt et al., (1993). It involves looking at:

1   The initial scope for change at the four hospital sites in our study (Tilley et al., 1991);

2   The purchasing process, in particular the purchasing strategies of the main NHS commissioners of these provider units and how they emerge (Tilley and Salt 1994);

3   The provider strategies of the hospital units (Baeza et al., 1993);

4   Inter and intra professional relations in our hospitals -this being the focus of the current chapter.

The examination of professional relations conducted in the chapter will proceed in three basic directions:

1   Given the degree of change involved, the starting point is to look at the implementation process and organizational power. The health Reforms have introduced a separation between purchasers, the district health authorities (DHAs) and the GP fundholders (GPFHs), and the now dominant type of provider, the NHS trust, and associated with this, the creation of a quasi market in health care services. The latter has considerably more significance in London and the other large cities where there is at least an element of contestability if not often competition in the strong sense of the word. The chapter offers an outcomes approach by putting the stress on contracts won by and resources available (beds, clinical staffing, budgets) to different medical specialties within hospitals. Attention will centre on important instances where disjunctions occur, i.e., contracts and resources do *not* move in sympathy. Furthermore, an emphasis on disjunctions puts the spotlight on resistance to change as the disjunctions scrutinized in the chapter flow from major intentions of the policy makers.

2   From a fieldwork standpoint there are various phases in identifying and exploring such disjunctions. The chapter will proceed using the outcomes approach, partially as data from only some of these will be offered at this stage in the research work.

3   The chapter will conclude by beginning to draw the threads together in the form of two questions:
a) Does the material presented in 2 above add to our understanding of the nature of disjunctions?

b) Even in the preliminary analysis of disjunctions offered here, it has been necessary to have some knowledge of the hospital's basic strategic position and response to that. At this stage is it possible to reach any conclusions about such factors, relations between senior consultants, the medical school and general management, and the effect of these on the level of disjunctions experienced in particular units?

The Government's current health policies are sufficiently radical and affect a public service of such prominence that there are available a considerable number of studies of what they involve (e.g. Butler, 1992; Harrison et al., 1992; Appleby, 1992; Tilley, 1993; and Drummond et al., 1993) even though there is much less detail on the actual implementation processes. Readers unfamiliar with the basic parameters of the current health policy should refer to these accounts.

From all of them it is clear that the Reforms are intended to change activities, professional relations and the major structures of the Service. All of this is likely to increase the degree of organizational politics in and around hospitals, and thence its likely value in understanding the implementation process.

The implementation process and organizational power

Seeing organizations as 'politically negotiated orders' (Bacharach and Lawler, 1980, p.1) is now well acknowledged, especially among UK writers. Even in ordinary times not only can internal power relations be exercised in ways that have consequences for 'resource allocations, administrative succession, structures, and strategic choices' (Pfeffer, 1981, p. 231) but also the scope for organizational change - the central focus of the Greenwich work on NHS hospitals - is affected by 'the history of attitudes and relationships between interest groups in and outside' the organization (Pettigrew, 1985, p. 27). These interest groups include the politicians, the DoH and the the NHS Executive; RHAs and the outposts; DHAs and other purchasers; and the acute providers, their major occupational and professional groupings.

This section will concentrate on two issues:

1 How to detect and study the workings of power and influence at the hospital level whilst the Reforms are implemented? By concentrating on the *outcomes* of power chiefly in the form of disjunctions between contracts won by particular specialties and the resources they are able to command, it is possible to gauge the extent to which old power centres hold onto past gains and frustrate the change process.

2 Developing the idea of disjunction, in particular, which types of disjunctions will be stressed in the current chapter.

When looking at the implementation of the health Reforms from inside acute hospitals, this chapter is concerned largely with different specialties within hospitals with differing degrees of power and influence. A key question is whether such power and influence can be deployed in ways which substantially affect whether the intentions of the policy makers actually prevail at the hospital level. Further, at a time of large scale change in the Health Service, organizational power is likely to be more 'dense' and vigorously applied and therefore ought to constitute a central focus for organizational researchers.

Whether all this is true is ultimately an empirical question. However, it is not difficult to find support for such views in the literature. For instance, Pettigrew, who has been influential in ensuring that British organizational analysis is well aware of the workings of power, makes similar points. First, 'politics in organizations breed in *times of change*' (1985, p. 43, emphasis added) as old and new power centres jostle with one another to maintain and expand their influence. Second and related to this, Pettigrew (1983, p. 107) talks about the likely 'persistence of centres of power in the transition from rich to poor'. The first factor is affecting all NHS institutions. As the Greenwich research project is based on an examination of four NHSTs, three of which are in London and are mainly facing a shrinking resource cake, the second point is also of clear significance to these hospitals and also many others in large cities.

Reflecting on Pettigrew's two statements it is clear that a key issue has to do with managing transitions, the winner and losers that arise from organizational change, and the pressure on our hospitals to engage in the painful process of taking out fixed costs, including staff: who should lose and by how much?

Pettigrew further suggests that 'political processes evolve at the group level from the division of work in the organization' (1975, p. 192). In a multi professional organization like the NHS this should direct attention not only to relations between professions but also within them. Despite this, some earlier accounts of the Reforms seem disposed to overly stress inter professional relations, particularly the straight doctors versus general managers picture (e.g. Strong and Robinson, 1990) to the neglect of the intra professional ones.

Despite Griffiths (1983) and the more recent Reforms, NHS hospitals remain largely what Mintzberg (1983, p. 165) terms professional bureaucracies. The pecking order, both between and within professions, is a key factor influencing what actually emerges when implementing large scale change. The research evidence (for instance, Rosoff and Leone, 1991) suggests a relative stability to the public's prestige ratings of different specialties within medicine. However, the concern in this chapter needs to be rather different; the focus must be firmly placed on what Pettigrew (1985) calls 'power in possession'. Thus, for example, it is such things as 'the motivation, resources and skills' (Haugaard, 1992, p. 14) that exist and are deployed by actual professional groupings and sub groupings in particular hospitals to support or resist the implementation of a particular policy that are important.

One way of proceeding is to focus precisely on the likely 'persistence of centres of power' mentioned above by Pettigrew and the probability that, when implementing a new policy, the transitions are unlikely to be particularly smooth affairs. Those who might be clear winners, if the intent of the policy makers were to fully prevail, may find their winnings curtailed or eliminated because those who created their empires in easier times and/or under earlier policies may be able to mobilize power to retain their relative privilege or at least limit their own losses. If this occurs to a significant degree, it will be termed here a disjunction. This concept is of central importance for the rest of the chapter.

Which disjunctions?

When Government ministers were promoting the NHS Reforms, they often repeated the health version of a dictum used in most areas of public services where the Conservatives have sought significant change. In the health services sphere it was rendered as 'money will follow the patient'. However, precisely what this means in terms of the details of the health Reforms is not easy to discern.

It certainly does not have much meaning at the literal level. Perhaps it can be given practical import by relating it to the change of the NHS funding formula to a weighted capitation basis by the policy makers? Except in the case of GP fundholding (purchasers who are still likely to be funded on a referral basis), the new formula for DHA funding largely reflect the number of residents within the authorities' catchment areas. The DoH and the RHA top slice such funds for various reasons before they reach the DHA. Although this might well produce disjunctions, the focus in this chapter is on disjunctions within hospitals.

The logic of the internal market requires that the resources flowing to different specialties should be connected to the contracts or service agreements for such specialties. Significant instances where this is not the case are prima facie instances of disjunction. Not only may they reveal important things about the inner workings of power within the hospital but also the ending of such disjunctions could be seen as one way of giving meaning to the notion that 'money will follow the patient'. In theory the task of eliminating large existing disjunctions and ensuring new ones do not arise should ultimately rest with the hospital's general management. As the remainder of the chapter begins to show, their actual role may be quite different.

Four different types of disjunction will be considered in this chapter. They emerge because the linkage that ought to exist between contracts awarded and either workloads actually achieved or resources used is clearly and significantly broken:

Linkage 1 (L1) disjunctions arise where the workloads actually achieved in a particular specialty vary significantly from the level of finished consultant episodes[1] (FCEs) specified in the contracts. Thus, L1 disjunctions are output disjunctions; all the remaining ones are resource disjunctions.

L2 disjunctions occur where beds allocated and/or clinical staff numbers working in a specialty do not respond to changes in the levels of contracts won by the specialty.

L3 disjunctions result where the specialty's budget allocation likewise does not react to variations in the contracts awarded.

L4 disjunctions emerge where the specialty under or overspends its budget allocation.

This is presented diagrammatically in Figure 7.1 A number of points should be made. First, only the numbered linkages, and possible disjunctions, shown in Figure 7.1 will be discussed. The two unnumbered linkages will be ignored as they are likely to be less important and significantly dependent on the four that are covered.

Second, although it has already been observed that it is important to see disjunctions at the individual specialty level, they are clearly linked to whole hospital factors like the unit's overall strategy and relations with the external world more generally. For example, the DoH has a policy to cut junior doctors' hours.

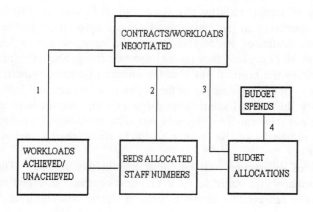

Figure 7.1   **Workloads and resource flows in specialties**

While 'external' to the particular hospital, it is clearly going to affect staff numbers and budgets and thence potentially L2-4. What are inner hospital factors in terms of the limits set in this chapter carry both their own local histories and much wider histories too or, as Meyer and Scott (1992, p. 16) put it 'institutional environments are notoriously invasive'.

Third, some of the four linkages, for instance, budget allocations and spends (L3 and L4) which may give rise to disjunctions could be closely related to one another. However, for analytical purposes it is useful to treat each separately even though, when presenting some of the field material in the next section, it may be convenient to consider both in the one discussion. A budget overspend, which if it continues and is large enough would constitute a significant L4 disjunction, might lead next year to a cut in allocation (L3). In this case all the material will be considered under L3 simply because it first arises in terms of L3.

Fourth, some linkages may appear too similar conceptually to warrant distinguishing. Given that the pay of clinical staff working in a specialty is the dominant item in its budget statement (as it is still likely to be produced), it may seem that budget allocations (L3) and beds allocated/staff numbers (L2) to contracts awarded are not too different. However, typically they are prepared by different professions - the budget by accountants and others in finance and staff numbers by clinical managers. Each is likely to be using different criteria and in this case to merge the two would be to lose something potentially significant.

Having established the linkages and possible output and resource disjunctions, how can relevant data be produced to explore them?

Using the outcomes approach, partially

This section has three aims:

1 To consider the various data gathering phases and methods that are used to produce data on disjunctions in the full Greenwich hospital study and indicate what part of this will be reported in this chapter.

2 To describe very briefly the four hospitals participating in the Greenwich study.

3 To begin to present some results from particularly the first phase of the full Greenwich analysis. This is designed to partially explore whether there are major disjunctions at work at the four hospitals sites and begin to understand something of how they function.

Different phases of identifying dislocations

As the Greenwich University study of disjunctions proceeds, it is passing through a number of phases and using a variety of approaches and methods. The reason for these different phases and methods is to be able compare, verify and develop the results of one research strategy in relation to another. The full analysis is still being conducted.

But, as the Greenwich University team are developing it, an outcomes approach to organizational change is not only concerned with the mere existence or otherwise of disjunctions. Although, due to its different aims, the Greenwich research brings in 'process issues' less and at a different time than NHS managers and management consultants actually involved in promoting change in their hospitals, such issues are not ignored. However, the outcomes approach derives much of its distinctiveness precisely by *starting* with end results and then working back to social context, including some of the processes, involved.

There are real practical problems for researchers, as opposed to change managers, proceeding in what might otherwise seem to be a straight line. To study what is happening in *all* specialties and work through to the outcomes is an unnecessarily daunting task for researchers to undertake. It is ruled out by the sheer size and the number of specialties involved.

The outcomes approach focuses attention only on those specialties who, judged by the results they are able to obtain, are resisting key parts of the health Reforms as publicly enunciated by the policy makers. This is so because the four disjunctions defined earlier were derived straight from the declared policy intentions of the politicians, particularly those to do with the creation of a quasi health care market.

Thus, resistance to change is clearly a central feature of the outcomes approach. However, if some change practitioners like to imagine such resistance largely as produced by individuals, the Greenwich team is focusing the attention elsewhere, at the specialty or occupational level.

To only identify significant disjunctions and little else would be rather barren and uninteresting. Having identified important disjunctions, the Greenwich team will, certainly in the full programme of research, devote considerable effort to understanding their histories, social and strategic contexts, and the tactics and meanings ascribed by key figures in the specialties that benefit from such disjunctions (dubbed 'winning' specialties in this chapter) and those disadvantaged by them ('losing' specialties).

This full programme of research has five phases.

1   The commencing phase is derived largely from the team and the knowledge of the hospital and some of the disjunctions at work it has already identified on the basis of the field work carried out. This knowledge is not inconsiderable as the Greenwich research team had already been at work for over two years before it came to focus major attention on internal disjunctions. Considerable numbers of key personnel had been interviewed, management and clinical meetings observed, questionnaires administered, and health authority and hospital documents gathered, examined and analyzed (Salt et al., 1993). It was, in fact, from this work that the idea of disjunctions as a reseach focus partly arose.

The field work material reported on later in the section mainly derives from this first source.

2   The next phase, the key informant phase, is to ask key informants whether major disjunctions exist in their hospitals. The purpose is to refine the work from the commencing phase and discover more of how significant disjunctions work. These informants have come to light during the course of research work conducted to date. They are people high enough in the organizational hierarchy and possessing the requisite analytical skills to possess a much broader knowledge of the hospital than most of its many employees have.

3   The next step is a statistical phase: to seek apparently significant disjunctions on the basis of an examination of relevant statistics about contracts, beds, staffing and budgets.

4   The ground is then prepared for a major interviewing phase. From the first and second phases the team is deriving a list of individuals who could provide much more detailed information about disjunctions. This material is designed to confirm, elaborate or refute what has already been tentatively established and reported in the current chapter. The interviewers will also be seeking an understanding of the history and social context surrounding important disjunctions. As suggested earlier in this sub-section, this includes a grasp of:

a)   The broader strategic context and response in which they occur.

b)   The tactics deployed by winning and losing specialties in directly producing dislocated outcomes.

c)   An understanding of the social meaning winners, losers and others attach to major disjunctions. This would include general management, the medical director, the medical school, the DHA and community health council (CHC).

In other words, if disjunctions are the outcome of power successfully exercised within hospitals (but usually reliant on resources, symbolic and otherwise, beyond it), there is a need to understand as far as possible the social production of the disjunction particularly as it takes place within the hospital but also with some understanding of its external reference points.

5   Clearly the major interviewing phase will be the most time consuming, labour intensive part of the research work. However, it is good practice e.g. (Willis 1980) to have a final feedback phase. Given the nature of hospital timetabling arrangements for clinical staff, the feedback planned will be of a limited nature. The team will take back to key informants the main findings that have emerged to this point and ascertain their validity and make any necessary alterations.

The key informants will not only be those involved in the commencing phase but also could emerge in other phases. Further, they will also include people with different areas of expertise. The reason for this is that properly analysing organizational disjunctions is a complex matter. It is unclear what a 20 per cent increase in contracts should mean if it were to fully flow through to the budget allocation of a specialty (L3) and thence not give rise to a disjunction. Such concerns will be returned to when L3 disjunctions are discussed below. However, the problem is not an overwhelming one as the concern in this chapter is with significant disjunctions with a clear impact on intra or inter professional relations. If a 20 per cent increase in contracts were accompanied by no rise, or even a noticeable cut, in a specialty's budget that should be investigated.

Before the Reforms there were no data available to establish L3 disjunctions or any other sort of disjunctions as defined here. Not only were hospital information systems inadequate managerially but also it is only the existence of the contracting system that has enabled their identification by outside analysts, even if the process is complex and difficult. But for such outsiders there is still no way to assess the adequacy of the base line figures.

In other words, the idea of disjunction available to independent researchers is a *relative, not absolute*, one. It is only possible to ascertain what change has occurred since the Reform, not whether the base line figures are fair. Insiders are not in the same position. For example, it is entirely possible for the finance department to carry out its own research as to what an adequate base line budget for a specialty is. They then could identify absolute disjunctions. Of course politically such zero based budgeting might be assailed by vested interests in hospitals as it has in the private sector. Interestingly enough some NHS hospital managements are themselves beginning to analyze resource flows in disjunction terms similar to those discussed in the chapter. The internal market does introduce a greater degree of transparency and, in theory, ought to encourage not only researchers but also management to think in these terms. In this particular chapter the data reported below derives essentially from the commencing phase although, as information is beginning to come in on the second and third phases, it will be used where appropriate. Consequently, all the chapter really aims to establish is the utility of the idea of output and resource disjunctions and some initial, broad ideas about how they work. However, the full meaning of a concept is related to all the ways in which it will be operationalized. In other words, the preliminary report offered in this chapter needs to be seen in the context of the entire exercise currently underway to fully investigate disjunctions.

After very briefly describing the four provider units in the study, some of the preliminary results will be considered.

The four hospitals in the Greenwich study

In the order the team started data gathering, the NHS providers are:

1 The only district general hospital (DGH) of the four, London District Trust (LDT)[2], a third wave NHS Trust.

2 Inner London Trust (ILT), a large teaching hospital, that was a first wave trust.

3 Midlands City Trust (MCT), another teaching hospital, which acquired trust status in 1992.

4 South London Trust (SLT), also a teaching hospital, which like LDT became a trust in 1993.

The material presented in the balance of this section particularly concerns the years 1992-93 to 1993-94.

As was said at the outset, the chapter only considers acute hospital providers and focuses on the inner London teaching hospital. This influenced the type of hospital involved in the study and the degree of depth to which research was carried out. Thus, the centre piece of the entire Greenwich study of the Reforms is a detailed comparision of ILT and SLT. Less attention is being paid to LDT and MCT. Their inclusion is chiefly to place the main comparison between the two London teaching hospitals in a wider setting. These choices are particularly evident in the full scale study of disjunctions which is only being undertaken at ILT and SLT.

L1 disjunctions between contracted and achieved workloads

Although some may see it as part of a rationing process, in policy terms the creation of the internal market ought to be accompanied by hospital providers ensuring that they match actual with contracted workloads. Any work that is over the contracted target will not be paid for by the purchaser and thence the provider unit has to cover the cost of that additional work out of its own resources. Thus, L1 disjunctions are likely to strain already tight resources and lead to robbing Peter to pay Paul situations - but the losing Peter tends to be the less specialized services like general surgery, general medicine, psychiatry and health care for the elderly (HCE) rather than the high tech, glamorous services such as renal, liver and cardiac services, oncology, and neurosciences.

From the Greenwich research large disjunctions between work done and contracted workloads existed at all hospitals being studied. Understanding L1, like the other three linkages, requires some knowledge of the environment providers' (Baeza et al., 1993) and purchasers' (Tilley and Salt, 1994) function in and the major strategic choices they make. In order to shorten the discussion, the initial focus will be on the total L1 disjunction ILT as a whole faced. Given that linkages and disjunctions as defined here essentially work at the specialty level, some analysis will then be offered at a degree of disaggregation below the whole unit level for ILT before briefly comparing and contrasting their experience with that at the three other sites.

In 1991-92 when the internal market was operating under steady state, ILT went nearly 4 per cent over its contracted activity level. ILT top management did not present this 'over activity' or 'over production' as a problem but rather as an intentional strategy. Although the Trust managed to fund this over activity out of its own resources in 1991-92, the disjunction became a real problem in the 1992-93 contract negotiations with the local purchaser. ILT management wanted the DHA to contract for the actual workloads of the previous year, including the extra 4 per cent but at higher prices which would have pushed up the total bill by 8 per cent. It was the DHA's refusal, or inability, to comply which forced ILT to try and match their activity to the contracting levels that were eventually negotiated for 1992-93.

The compromise agreement that was eventually reached involved concessions from the DHA as well as the provider. At that stage ILT, unlike many other NHSTs, covered both acute and community services and this probably increased the frustrations the DHA faced in achieving its priorities - themselves being part of the Government's declared policy in *Health of the Nation* (DoH, 1991) -of increasing its community contracts while the acute sector was working over contract. Certainly significant L1 disjunctions in acute services at ILT highlight the different objectives between provider management and their purchasers who have overall responsibility for health commissioning.

NHS managers have never found it easy to control their doctors' activity and so, although the ILT management presented the over activity as a conscious decision to enable them to be in a strong position for the 1992-93 contracting round, this seems more a rationalization of matters not fully within their control. LDT adopted a similar stance to that of ILT and one that perhaps further undermines the conscious strategy interpretation. In this case managers interviewed said that a conscious decision was taken in November 1992 to overshoot contracts. The main reason given for this was again that it would supposedly strengthen their position with the purchasers. As with ILT, this turned out to be a somewhat naive view and perhaps reflects the limited experience at that time of the contracting system..

However, at LDT this strategy seriously backfired in two respects. First, LDT actually lost some contracts, for example, in ophthamology to neighbouring provider units largely because the purchaser was dissatisfied with the quality of the local provision and surprisingly (Tilley and Salt, 1994) could not obtain the changes it required. Second, in line with Government policy, their purchasers insisted that LDT make 2 per cent 'efficiency savings' in 1993-94 (Appleby and Little, 1993), not on their contracted workload for 1992-93 but on their higher outturn figures.

As already indicated, this sub section works largely at the whole unit level. However, as not all of ILT's specialties had L1 disjunctions, moving briefly to the specialty level will assist understanding. The renal and cardiology departments kept strictly to contract but theirs are low volume, high cost procedures - and thence relatively easy to accurately track. They have rudimentary cost and volume contracts which, given the life and death nature of the work done, are renegotiated with the purchasers when the trigger is reached. In contrast ILT's general surgery certainly did not hold to contracts but their work was on block contracts and much more of the high volume, low cost variety - which was therefore much more difficult to track.

What additional factors might explain the surgery dislocation and the over runs more generally? First, there was the background factor that in the first year of implementation and in the run up to the 1992 election, and beyond, the Government was very keen to see NHSTrusts in particular doing more work. For instance, the NHS(M)E (1991, p. 4) reported a 3.7 per cent increase in activity countrywide after the first six months of the Reforms. However, it is already apparent from the ILT case that there can be costs for such increases. Second, both GPs and hospital doctors wanted to treat more patients, even when not encouraged. Some may have positively not wanted to fit in with the new contracting system. Third, a few may have felt less secure in the new NHS world and increased their own workloads to strengthen personal position.

With our second London teaching hospital, SLT, the general story was also one of 'over activity' on contracted targets as at ILT and LDT. During 1992-93 SLT as a whole dealt with 5 per cent more FCEs than the previous year. General management put half this figure down to 'better recording of activity'. They also studied the two specialties most over target to ascertain the financial effects of the higher than commissioned activity levels. They identified the two largest areas of activity in the Hospital, surgery and medicine, as the main 'culprits'. From internal documents it is clear that the net effect of the 'excess' activity costs was around £250,000 -300,000. This was a crucial concern for SLT senior management as the whole hospital had a deficit in 1992-93 of around £500,000 and this could have endangered their efforts to become a full NHST at the start of 1993-94.

As most of this 'excess' occurred in the surgical directorate, the financial implications of not controlling the 'over activity' are self evident. All the factors that produced this will only emerge from the full five part data gathering and analysis outlined earlier. But, and this will become increasingly important as the present section proceeds, *senior management* quite consciously encouraged cardiology and neurosciences in particular to greatly overshoot their contracts.

This story will be returned to as later disjunctions are considered and in the concluding section. At this stage it is sufficient to say management's purpose in encouraging this 'over production' was to bolster cardiology and neurosciences' position. The Specialty Reviews following Tomlinson (1992) suggested they should be moved from SLT to a neighbouring teaching hospital.

The same broad picture of 'excess production' is also true of MCT, the only out of London hospital in the study. Although in 1992-93 they were in total nearly three per cent over their contracted target, interestingly enough this was not presented by management as a problem. However, they operate in a different internal market from the other three hospitals; in London competition is real, if limited, in its extent. There was no competition between MCT and its nearest neighbour. Moreover, unlike hospitals in London and other large cities, it was not subject to any of the restructuring moves outlined at the beginning of the chapter.

In sum then, given that the disjunction work from the Greenwich team has not passed through all its phases, it is not possible yet to fully disaggregate to the specialty level. Until this is fully done, it is not possible to know precisely which specialties continue to exceed and which under achieve contracts over significant time periods and why. However, what is already apparent as the work is being undertaken is that, the more specialized services, ILT's renal and cardiology specialties were almost the exception rather than the rule in keeping to their contracted levels. Speaking more broadly and over the four hospitals such high tech, glamour services were often amongst the 'worst offenders' in terms of L1 disjunctions and delivering these higher workloads is of itself likely to increase their L2-4 resource disjunctions . Furthermore, as the managements at the four sites, especially the three London ones who faced considerable financial stringency, became more concerned about 'over production' the only specialties they could easily press into reducing their activities tended to be the historically weak ones. This might even involve management requiring them to keep their outturn below the contracts they are supposed to be meeting. This was what happened to health care for the elderly at SLT despite it being an emergency based service for highly vulnerable patients.

L2 disjunctions between contracted workloads and the allocation of beds and staff

Traditionally beds have been jealousy guarded by consultants, their allocation often being determined on historical grounds. If the Reforming NHS, certainly the London Health Service, is functioning within a quasi market, there is a clear need to link contracted workloads to the allocation of beds.

A host of seemingly quite technical factors are involved, e.g. different bed turnover rates, indivisibilities, complementaries, and so forth as well as other factors with a more obvious social content such as the influence of medical schools in teaching hospitals over bed levels. There is in reality no such thing as a purely technical factor in this or any other area; they are always socially constructed even if also possessing technical dimensions.

Furthermore, as with disjunctions in the L1 area, frequently L2 type disjunctions can only be properly appreciated if there is also some grasp of the strategic context in which they arose.

With this in mind, the discussion returns to SLT's general surgery specialty which, as was mentioned in the previous sub-section, substantially overran its 1992-93 contracts. Although this had adverse financial implications for the Hospital as a whole, a question arises as to how this increased activity was actually accommodated given that the number of beds used by this directorate actually fell.

Furthermore, to what extent did this give rise to a disjunction and to what extent did it involve other factors?

The first way surgery accommodated its increased workload was through SLT's policy, vigorously backed up by their main purchaser, of increasing the proportion of surgery undertaken in their new day case surgery centre. This has risen from about 10 per cent in 1991 to 40 per cent by the end of the 1993-94 financial year. Thus, it may seem there is no real disjunction as defined earlier in this chapter but simply an adjustment arising from technological advance.

However, this was not the only factor that led to general surgery's bed losses. In particular, as was indicated in the discussion of L1 disjunctions, management wanted to expand a regional specialty - cardiology - and thence this specialty was allowed to take beds from surgery. The stated managerial aim was to build up one discipline at the expense of the other. In other words, part of general surgery's bed loss is a clear and significant L2 disjunction and one facilitated by general management's own action.

At LDT both surgery and ophthamology lost contracts and thence beds and capacity. However, the fall in the number of ophthamology beds was not as great as indicated by the fall in contracted workload. Senior management at the Hospital claimed this too was part of a deliberate strategy, in this case because management believed the bed loss would be too great to be implemented all at once. Whether what was involved here was simply a time lag in fully cutting bed numbers or a significant disjunction is hard to settle at this stage. Its development needs to be watched and perhaps some knowledge sought of LDT's past history in terms of bed cuts.

L2, as presented in Figure 7.1, has a second aspect: the linkage or otherwise between contracts and clinical staffing levels. As already indicated, the different types of linkages and disjunctions are often related to one another. If L1 disjunctions can give rise to L2 disjunctions, the converse is also true. In this case, if significant contract/staffing disjunctions are allowed to arise, the failure to cut capacity could mean 'over production'. This is so because medical staff numbers, along with the number of beds capacity, largely determine the level of clinical activity (van Doorslaer and van Vliet, 1989). Therefore if the number of contracts goes down, the logic of the new system calls for a reduction in the number of clinical staff unless this situation is thought to be temporary, e.g. replacement contracts are likely to be forthcoming before long.

Throughout the NHS, certainly from 1993-94 and onwards, skill mix reviews of nursing, market testing of non clinical functions and significant redundancies in both areas are increasingly the order of the day. New types of job, frequently outside of Whitley categories and scales, are being created as well as the introduction of rising numbers of health care assistants to replace the much smaller numbers of nursing auxiliaries. The latter development is made possible by the major change in nurse education implied by Project 2000. All this complicates the analysis of Linkage 2. With many hospitals facing difficult financial situations, certainly including the ones in this study, human resource management is emerging as a significant area for achieving cost reductions (Salt, 1994). Furthermore, although the discussion here is in terms of the linkage or otherwise between contracts and staffing, such industrial relations developments are *not* necessarily restricted to specialties which are losing contracts.

The group that to date have been left out of all these major, frequently painful, developments, is doctors and consultants. This is true in relation to the four hospitals in the Greenwich study but it goes far beyond this. For instance, at ILT, although general surgery lost two whole wards and a number of nurses, it did not lose any medical staff. Given that such situations are not isolated events but occurring increasingly, they are a major, present day illustration of the relative power of the medical profession compared with that of nurses, and, for that matter, all other NHS professions and occupations. One senior ILT manager remarked:

> we have never lost doctors. Management can't do that; we are too wimpish.
> The honest answer is that we failed (to reduce the number of doctors even if
> their contracts fall significantly). The top management isn't strong enough to
> take out the doctors.

Not all ILT general managers interviewed presented the situation in general surgery in such stark terms. Some wanted to link the failure to reduce the number of surgeons to longer term strategic considerations. Such managers suggested the reduction in contracts for general surgery was a temporary situation and, once the reorganization of London's acute services was complete, the contract levels for surgery at ILT should rise. From this perspective a reduction in the number of medical staff would be unwise when doctors would be needed in the long term. But such comments are silent about the differential treatment of doctors, and nurses and other occupations.

SLT provides a further example of an L2 disjunction between contracts and staffing levels with the same inter professional dimension to it. As at ILT, the expressed managerial aim was revealed in internal documents as 'reducing surgery's capacity'. But in neither case has there been any attempt to reduce the number of surgeons. Likewise at LDT, although surgery contracts have been reduced, the directorate had not lost any surgeons or other medical staff. However, the number of nurses on those wards has been cut and the use of agency staff stopped altogether.

Overall by 1992-93 in the hospitals in this study clear inter professional differences in the treatment of doctors and nurses were opening up. The Government's commitment to reducing junior doctors hours, but without allocating substantial new funds, furthers this process. In later years the differential treatment of doctors and nurses has become more pronounced with many specialties having to reduce costs by 'down sizing' irrespective of their contract position.

The medical school might also have a significant influence on L2 linkages between contract levels, and both beds and staff numbers. One MCT consultant indicated that the school could be a powerful ally either when reductions in beds or staff were threatened or when a consultant wanted to make a case for an increase in beds or staff. Further, the Royal Colleges have guidelines concerning the number of beds and medical staff they deem necessary and the university to which the medical school belongs might also be mobilized or at least management fear this may occur. At the four hospitals in the Greenwich study the medical director is the only senior manager trained as a doctor. The rest, lacking medical credentials and legitimacy, could hardly welcome interventions from any of these quarters.

The role of the medical school, its relations with the different specialties and with general management clearly is of major importance in teaching hospitals. It is something that will be singled out for discussion at the end of the chapter. Of major importance is which specialties might gain in disjunction terms from the interaction between the main specialties, the medical school and general management?

L3 disjunctions between contracted workloads and budget allocations

There are various seemingly quite technical problems that could tend to complicate clear identification of true L3 dislocations. On the surface the problems appear to be merely accounting ones. Two of these will be considered in an effort to demonstrate that, as with L2 (contracts to beds/staffing), such technical accounting problems have important social implications too, including affecting the level of disjunctions.

The first of these relates to so called 'efficiency savings'. During the years particularly focused on the Government has imposed such efficiency savings on all NHS hospitals effectively cutting their overall budget allocation. Moreover, local efficiency savings might also be applied. Thus, for instance, in 1993-94 SLT specialties faced 4 per cent budget reductions, half imposed nationally and the other half locally.

As is common practice throughout the Health Service, SLT proceeded to reduce the existing budgets of all specialties by 4 per cent. On the surface this may seem the only fair way of proceeding. However, given that each specialty has a different cost structure, i.e. different proportions of variable, fixed, semi fixed and semi variable costs, blanket reductions can introduce new disjunctions or increase existing ones even if, on the face of it, the policy seems to suggest otherwise. A more sophisticated approach which takes into account important differences in cost behaviour is not yet possible because, SLT (and for that matter NHS hospitals generally, including the other three hospitals studied) are not particularly advanced in analysing costs.

Such distortions do *not* fall randomly. Some of the more specialised services (e.g. cardiac and oncology services) have a higher level of variable costs and thence more scope to reduce costs. The less specialised services (say, HCE and psychiatry) have mainly fixed (staffing) costs, which by definition are largely unavoidable in the short term, and therefore more seriously affected by across the board budget cuts. Moreover, the latter services tended to lose, or lose more, with respect to the earlier disjunctions as well and have a long history of relative disadvantage.

Another seemingly technical accounting problem that causes difficulties in even identifying real disjunctions between contracted workloads and budget allocations is that the allocation of costs to budgets is still quite rudimentary at the four hospitals considered in this chapter. Again in this they are in no way untypical of NHS hospitals generally.

Although changes are beginning to occur, specialty budget statements at the four hospitals during 1992-93 - 1993-94 mainly conformed to the old GL4 statement. This only covered what various departments spend on pay (narrowly defined as medical and nursing staff only) and non pay items (mainly restricted to those consumables directly used in the department). The costs of back up staff and support staff such as portering and hotel services, and even the costs of central management or IT, need to be included. Additionally, capital charges on resources used and credits like the Service Increment for Teaching and Research (SIFTR) were not yet allocated to user specialties. The former omission again is likely to work in favour of the more high tech specialties who tend to use far greater capital assets than the less specialized services.

However, the Greenwich team has seen plenty of evidence that the situation is changing. Perhaps then this only constitutes a temporary problem. For instance, by the end of the 1993-94 financial year, SLT management had plans to include the costs of patient services, pathology and the like on clinical budgets. Based on historical usage levels these budgets were beginning to be devolved down to individual specialties who would then be held responsible for managing that budget. In line with national developments, SLT, and the other three hospitals, are beginning the costly move towards creating an 'internal market' within hospitals between internal providers of services and the purchasing specialties.

As these become operational, it would be an interesting research question to study the details of how the new transfer pricing systems work. For instance, how are prices being calculated and will specialties be able to chose between internal and external suppliers? This is another area where the seeming mechanics of another type of accounting device can have significant social implications (Mehafdi, 1991) and potentially produce disjunctions.

Nonetheless, there are other pressures encouraging the move towards fully comprehensive budget statements which do not omit significant costs. For example, increasing numbers of NHS hospitals, including the hospitals in the study, are finding it absolutely necessary to successful *purchasing negotiations* that they have a real idea of the cost of operating different specialties. This is opening up a gap between what is being done for purchasing (where all or most costs allocated) and internal budgeting purposes (where major costs still tend to be omitted). This gap in itself could constitute a lever encouraging change in the latter.

If so, that would undoubtedly constitute progress. However, it is hardly being unduly pessimistic to remind readers that the very process of allocating overheads is hardly trouble free! In fact, although private sector management accounting is lauded and increasingly deployed in the Reforming NHS, the whole area of apportioning such costs remains a *central* problem for managerial accountants in private companies (Johnson and Kaplan, 1987).

But beyond these two accounting problems which can affect disjunctions, what other L3 disjunctions is the research beginning to detect? Furthermore, is the L1 and L2 pattern of winners and losers reflected in the L3 area? The overall answer to this question is that the richer, more specialized services are indeed tending to become richer in budget terms too or, at minimum, bear less of the pain of cutbacks than the less specialized services.

This will be illustrated by looking, first, at ILT where one of the more specialised services (in this case renal) was not allowed to increase its budget in line with increasing contracts and, second, at SLT where a similar type of policy operated but to the disadvantage of the weaker specialties. The two cases illustrate important differences between SLT and the other three sites which will be considered in more detail in the next section.

As the Reforms are implemented, securing a favourable budget allocation (L3) is becoming more important than previously. In the past strong specialties tended to accept the budget allocation which was essentially just handed down to them by the finance department and likely to roll over the previous budget with adjustments for 'efficiency savings' and the like. However, the strong specialties knew there were few effective sanctions that could be imposed on the specialty itself if they overspent the allocation (L4). If there were casualties, they were in the managerial, not clinical ranks. In other words, unit general managers (UGMs) and other managers and accountants with large over spends might find themselves in trouble or even replaced by the local DHA.

This was something that successive policy changes, culminating in the current Reform package, were designed to check. By the start of the 1993 financial year SLT and LDT became NHS Trusts; ILT had become a first wave trust in 1991 and MCT the following year. They could no longer look to their home DHA to bail them out of such problems. As will soon become apparent in the discussion of L4 disjunctions, over spends do still arise but it is becoming increasingly difficult for most specialties in most NHS hospitals to ignore budgets with the impunity some did in the past. This is certainly the case with the three London hospitals in the study, particularly SLT and LDT, both of whom found themselves in particularly difficult funding situations.

What seems to be happening is that not only are budget negotiations between the specialties' senior clinicians, business managers and the like becoming more important but also both the speciality and general management/finance are thinking of specialties more as 'profit centres' than just 'cost centres' during budget negotiations even if this is not reflected in the hospital's organizational structure.

What then happened to ILT's renal department? Through an increase in contract income, the department saw itself ending 1992-93 earning a large revenue surplus for the Hospital and they very much wanted this extra income to flow through to them as an increase in budget allocation. This was hardly an unreasonable expectation in terms of the policy statements underlying the current Reform process. In fact, if this did not happen, it would, in the terms of this chapter, be an L3 disjunction. Initially renal's clinical director and other consultants understood that this was precisely what would happen; their 1993-94 budget allocation would be substantially increased to reward them for the increased contracts. They had already planned to use it on capital expenditure. As the budget negotiations proceeded, it became clear that general management had decided to change the rules originally enunciated and use much of this to support other services who had not fared as well in contract terms as renal.

This the ILT management group did in the name of 'corporate smoothing', something that is hardly unknown to private sector strategic decision making or, for that matter, other NHS hospitals. The justification in the NHS case is that the whole hospital had to survive and at the time ILT's overall strategic position was difficult. Redundancies and other cost cutting measures were going through.

Management used ILT's teaching status as a justification for changing the rules about contract surpluses and budgets and renal did, in fact, experience a significant L3 disjunction as a result. Although generally the relations between senior management and ILT's medical school were not especially close, the school supported the managers. Both argued that, if such contract losers were not helped, specialties could disappear which would seriously threaten the Hospital's teaching status. The renal department had little choice but to accept the need to support services that had lost contracts but they argued that this situation could not continue for long. Renal was strong enough to force general management to declare that in subsequent years much of the surplus from contracts would flow through into individual budget allocations.

The management have instituted, and have largely stuck to a new policy, which they dubbed 'internal brokerage'. While specialties that incur deficits may 'borrow' from other specialties, the finance department would adjust the new financial allocations to fully allow for this. The Hospital continued to face tight acute budgets. The new approach allows the Hospital as a whole to balance its books while still permitting individual services to keep 'surpluses' earned from contracts and compelling others to return 'debts' incurred.

According to senior management interviews at MCT, the out of London teaching hospital in the study, a similar policy of 'internal brokerage' applied there too. However, the finance interviews suggest the situation was more complex and far less clear cut than senior management had implied.

At precisely the same time that ILT's management conceded internal brokerage enabling renal to become an even stronger specialty in the Hospital's pecking order, SLT's managers were holding firmly to a corporate smoothing approach but in order to protect both their large specialties (medicine and surgery) and their more prestigious, specialized services at the obvious expense of the so called Cinderella ones. HCE, child health and physiotherapy were particularly affected. They were persuaded to under spend their 1992-93 budgets (L4 disjunction) in addition to having their budget allocations for 1993-94 decreased as well.

This was justified by a top SLT manager on the grounds that it was not 'strategically wise' to 'reign in certain over spenders yet' as the Specialty Reviews were then in progress and the management feared the outcome. The Reviews actually recommended that many of the more specialized services should be transferred out of SLT into a neighbouring hospital who would be left largely with the more routine services which would receive large contract increases. This outcome lead to senior management further strengthening the 'threatened', more specialized services which meant that their historically advantaged position was improved even more; they became even greater beneficiaries in terms of all the output (L1) and resource disjunctions (L2-4) considered in this chapter.

This was carried out with such consistency, and not only in the L3 area, and with senior consultants from the 'threatened' specialties, the medical school and general management working so closely together that SLT increasingly emerges as different from the ILT and MCT, the other two teaching hospitals in the study. Investigating this more fully is important and is something that will be returned to in the concluding section.

L4 disjunctions between budget allocations and spends

There can be many reasons for budget over and underspends. Efficiencies, inefficiencies, unrealistic budget allocations and changes in work practices are all examples of these. Clearly what is happening to budget allocations can have a noticeable effect on the actual level of expenditure. In the discussion of the former (i.e. L3 disjunctions) their interconnectedness has already emerged. However, given the importance of keeping spending by clinicians in check in earlier reforms and the current Reform package, separately discussing budgets and spend is worthwhile.

As for all the resource linkages and possible disjunctions, L4 disjunctions need to be seen in the light of the past history of the hospitals and the different specialties within them and their current strategic position. Even at this relatively early stage of the Greenwich study significant L4 disjunctions are emerging.

This was certainly the case at ILT, a first wave trust which somewhat unusually originally comprised both acute and community services. But by 1992-93 the two were being separated out and some would argue that L4 disjunctions were at the centre of that change.

In 1991-92 the overall community sector then within ILT underspent its budget by 1 per cent (nearly £300,000) and the acute sector had an overall overspend of four per cent (over £2 million.). Local GPs, none of whom were GPFHs and many of whom were opposed to the creation ILT as an NHS trust, claimed that a leaked Hospital document had informed the community services to underspend and thereby offset the acute overspend. There was much claim and counter claim around what actually occurred. Even among the managerial group the research team heard different views expressed.

Some managers seemed to accept at least an element of fault from their side in what the leading GPs portrayed as 'a raid on community resources'. Others offered more limited explanations, for example, arguing that the community services underspent because of problems faced in terms of staff recruitment and retention. There had been a Hospital wide recruitment freeze that had affected the community more than acute services. Such a view is silent as to why this was so and was allowed occur. Certainly the Greenwich fieldwork indicates that the influence of the acute services on ILT's general management was pervasive. The situation clearly reflects a major clash of priorities going beyond the confines of ILT. The purchasers wanted to move funding from acute to community services in line with their assessment of the needs of a local population comprising a large ethnic community and which the Director of Public Health saw as often ineffectively cared for by conventional hospital based medicine. This is quite consistent with the declared aims of national policy as set out in the DoH's *Health of the Nation* (1991).

The local DHA was a modest net gainer in terms of the change in the national funding formula in the Health Service. In the event extra funding was very slow emerging and until recently the DHA found it impossible to significantly increase community services. This shift was not helped by a trust management who were clearly much more deeply attuned to the needs of their strong but financially strapped acute sector. It is also worth remembering that in the discussion of Linkage 1 above, all four hospitals, including ILT, exceeded their acute contract levels which in ILT with its combined trust put real pressure on resources available to the community sector.

In the event the Tomlinson Inquiry (1992) required the breaking up of ILT into acute and community trusts. It appears that the ILT experience as a joint trust was a significant factor in the approach taken by both Tomlinson and the DoH to other joint trusts. For instance, SLT had to rapidly change their combined trust application into two. Interestingly LDT, the only DGH in the study, did emerge as a combined acute/community trust.

The type of budget situation ILT faced was not peculiar to it. At SLT, the other London teaching hospital considered here, it has already been indicated in the preceding sub section that HCE, child health and physiotherapy underspent their budgets because they were requested to and thereby offset overspending in other areas. As with ILT, the aim was to leave the entire hospital in a break even position 'at worst'.

MCT, the out of London teaching hospital studied, faced a much easier strategic position than either ILT or SLT. First, its DHA was a net gainer in capitation funding terms and, second, unlike SLT which was one of three large teaching hospitals in a small geographic area in London, MCT faced only one other hospital. Both hospitals agreed to continue the existing division of services in their relatively small city and the DHA largely went along with that situation (Baeza et al., 1993).

The much more relaxed context for MCT can be well illustrated in the L4 area. Its general surgery directorate had actually underspent the budget and used part of this to meet an overspend in theatres. As theatres had made a number of innovations important to surgery and which had resource implications not reflected in theatres 'somewhat unrealistic' budget figures, general surgery was prepared to fund theatres. This was subsequently institutionalized by finance when theatres' budget was officially increased and surgery's was adjusted downwards.

Beginning to pull the threads together

As already indicated, this chapter offers a preliminary analysis of the disjunction part of the overall Greenwich inquiry into the current Reforms and their organizational effects particularly on the large, famous inner London teaching hospital. It is preliminary as the overall data gathering plan has only been partly undertaken at this stage.

Readers may well want to reflect on what the chapter reveals about the validity of a comparative case study approach. Because the Greenwich work focused on the acute London teaching hospital, it is only likely to have clear relevance for hospitals undergoing similar experiences, i.e., other teaching hospitals and acute hospitals in large cities.

The case study approach clearly has weaknesses (for example, uncertain generalizability) as well as clear strengths (for instance, doing greater justice to the complexities involved in the implementation of the health initiatives). The latter is important because management and social science research into the implementation of the current health Reforms is still largely at the stage of discovery of knowledge rather than the verification of an already existing body of findings about implementing this major change in health policy. At the discovery stage the case study approach seems particularly appropriate. Given the surprisingly few studies of the organizational impact of implementing the Reforms (Tilley, 1993, Chapter 20), at least partial understanding can emerge.

Nonetheless, enough material has been presented even in this one chapter to be able to suggest that dislocations or disjunctions between contracts and actual workloads (L1) and between contracts and resource flows in specialties (L2-4), all things the Reformers want to eliminate, are still in existence at the four research sites between 1992-93 and 1993-94, and have increased over that period. Furthermore, the role general management have played in this process has at times been surprising and is something that this section needs to further clarify.

This concluding section will endeavour to pull together some of the significant preliminary threads by focusing in two directions:

1   To consider a few significant features that the chapter, especially the data about the hospitals, adds to understanding the nature of disjunctions.

2   A brief pulling together and adding to comments already made about strategic context, the type of relations between managers, consultants and the medical school, and its effects on disjunctions. Of particular interest is how changes in these factors affect the level and consistency of the disjunctions borne by the main losers, the less specialized services (e.g. surgery, HCE and psychiatry) and enjoyed by the chief beneficiaries, the more specialized, high tech glamour specialities (e.g. neurosciences, oncology, renal, cardiac).

On the Greenwich work and the nature of disjunctions

The chapter suggests that an outcomes approach can yield worthwhile results if the focus is not only on the results of the differential power of particular specialties but also something of the social context within which this is wielded. Social context in this single chapter has largely revolved around provider strategy and sketching something of the basically different strategic positions and responses the hospitals, especially ILT and SLT, operate in.

The full disjunctions approach being currently researched by the Greenwich team will enable more to be reported about the tactics, context, and history of such disjunctions.   It is further concerned with the social meanings 'winners' and 'losers' attach to significant disjunctions. Frequently for the high tech 'winners' this is being found to revolve particularly around the literally life and death circumstances in which they tend to operate. If one wanted to be unkind, one could say that shroud waving can pay dividends!

Even at this stage it is evident that the approach delivers more about intra rather than inter professional relations, i.e. it shows how one specialty and all the different types of staff associated with it are, in an NHS world of tight resources, gaining at the expense of another specialty and the various professionals that work in it.

There is no evidence of conscious decisions being made here to achieve health gain or cost effectiveness even though the policy makers say they want to see the NHS moving in this direction. Real movement down that path could require at minimum much more powerful DHAs than currently exist, armed with much more information than they currently have.

Both intra and inter professional relations can, and frequently do, pull in different directions. A key L2 disjunction discussed in the previous section related to the large numbers of nursing staff, rather than doctors, being made redundant as part of Government's moves to 'restructure' the London Health Service. Although a major inter professional difference, its impact varies with the particular specialty in which the nursing staff are working. Those operating within a strong, more specialized service are less likely to lose nurses than those in a weaker, less specialized department. Furthermore, there are likely to be many more nurses on higher grades in the former type of department than the latter, and the former are less likely to be affected by the skill mix reviews that are occurring in nursing throughout the country. Thus, cardiac services are likely to have many more G, H and I grade nurses than HCE; there will be significant numbers of A's in HCE but none in cardiac. The latter need to be more highly trained but again nursing skills are not just technical matters but are socially constructed as well (Smith, 1992; Crompton and Sanderson, 1990).

The London 'rationalization' moves and their impact on nurses are also instructive because contracts in the NHS internal market are hardly the only or even the main driver in this and many aspects of the Reforming NHS. It still remains largely politically driven from the centre, or centres - the politicians, DoH, including the NHSE and its outposts, and RHAs - even though some measure of local autonomy does exist for provider and purchaser managements (Tilley and Salt, 1994) to operate within. Meyer and Scott (1992) refer to this type of situation as 'fragmented centralization' and its importance becomes even clearer in the next and concluding sub section.

Basic provider strategy and disjunctions

It is already apparent that disjunctions form an important intersection point between inner and outer realities. How that intersection works and its impact on the level of disjunctions operating in hospitals is of major importance. Although a more considered view must await the full programme for studying disjunctions discussed earlier, some tentative points are beginning to emerge even from the preliminary work reported in this chapter. The task here is to briefly pull together the relevant material from the previous section and add any additional material needed to ensure clarity.

SLT is the appropriate starting point because it emerged from the previous section as rather different from the other three hospitals, including ILT, the other London teaching hospital in the study. More detail about its environmental circumstances and strategic responses is presented in Baeza et al. (1993), and Tilley and Salt (1994).

But in brief the following was involved. During 1992-93 and 1993-94 SLT's local health authority was a major net loser in the changeover to the new capitation funding arrangements. The number of hospitals in the area was considerable: apart from SLT, two famous teaching hospitals plus a district general hospital (DGH). Its original health authority had merged with two other authorities to reconstitute itself as a new, enlarged DHA. This body required each of the three teaching hospitals in the area to bear an equal share of the funding loss. Had this merger not occurred, SLT's share would have been much less. Furthermore, SLT had noticeably higher prices than its neighbouring hospitals. This was partly due to its longer than average bed stays and explains much of the adverse disjunctions for general surgery (e.g. the beds part of L2 above). In other words, they arose from deliberate managerial action to force general surgery and all the surgical specialties to adopt what management deemed to be more acceptable practices.

As the new DHA and the LIG Specialty Reviews saw it, the real solution to these woes required not only closure for one of SLT's neighbouring teaching hospitals but also SLT losing virtually all of its more specialized services to the other teaching hospital that would be left in the area. These specialties were precisely the ones that historically had the most privileged position in resource terms. Under these plans the less specialized side of the work at SLT would have benefited from huge increases in contracts.

General management, senior consultants from these historically privileged specialties, and the medical school all effectively came together to resist 'the super DGH threat'. These three groups united around what they defined as a severe crisis which was often articulated in terms of its possible implications for SLT's teaching status. Management cleared the way internally for the 'threatened specialties' to strengthen their position and hopefully thwart the DHA and LIG's plans for them as well as lobbying against them.

If it was thought that exceeding contracts (a L1 disjunction) would make any of the 'threatened specialties' harder to move to the neighbouring teaching hospital, SLT management permitted this and ensured that all the related linkages (L2-4) would operate strongly in their favour. Even if the specialty was losing contracts, it was allowed to have significant increases in all resource areas. In other words, as the Greenwich team moves towards the completion of the full disjunction analysis at SLT, a strong and entirely consistent pattern of winning by the more specialized services and losing by the others emerges. Given their overall funding situation, the consequences of the action stemming from this probably temporary 'alliance' of management, consultants from the high tech specialties and the medical school could do no other than significantly increase the existing disadvantage of the less specialized services.

Despite the DHA and the Specialty Reviews threatening to remove virtually all SLT's glamour services to another nearby teaching hospital, when the Secretary of State actually announced her decision she did not support these changes and SLT even made large gains in the threatened areas. Furthermore, around the same time the DHA concluded a renegotiation of capitation funding policy with its RHA which meant no further losses of funds for its hospitals. In dramatic fashion the crisis was over.

Does this mean SLT's crisis and how it was handled was no longer of relevance to understanding anything wider in the NHS? On the contrary, what happened in the crisis years is instructive, first, in terms of the temporary 'alliance' between three such powerful groups at SLT and, second, to contrast with the position at the other hospitals in the study, particularly ILT.

In general terms, it took serious external difficulties to push the three groups together. Their aim seems to have been the defence of the already dominant specialized services. As a consequence, general management - who in theory were the key change agents for the Reforms within the Hospital - was committed to supporting a major increase in these specialties favoured position in the Hospital. This was done in the name of responding to a 'crisis' of major proportions.

The same picture of severe crisis could not be said to exist at ILT, or MCT. What difference did this make? Virtually the same specialized services had occupied privileged positions prior to the current health Reforms. During 1992-93 and 1993-94 these specialties received general support from the medical school but not with quite the same vigour as at SLT. At both ILT and MCT both groups had much less close relations with general management than at SLT and they were punctuated by periods of dissension.

Without a 'crisis' to mobilize around, there was much less unity between the three groups and nothing of the coordinating and supporting role from management that gave rise to such a large and consistent increase in all four types of disjunctions at SLT. What appears to have happened is that the position of services like cardiology and renal in disjunction terms is much more patchy than at SLT. It even contains noticeable 'inconsistencies' in terms of which type of specialty gains or loses on individual disjunctions. Certainly compared with SLT the situation is much less in favour of the more specialized services and at the expense of the less specialized.

Nonetheless, the overall trend is still at least one of *relative* advantage for the high tech, glamour specialties. Thus, for instance, if there is a loss to be shared, the high tech specialties face less of the pain than the lower tech.

Notes

1. FCEs have been used because, as the team moved into gathering statistical information about disjunctions, it has not been able to obtain anything like full information on the monetary value of contracts awarded. However, as the key concern is with percentage changes, FCEs will still yield adequate results when the full disjunction analysis is available.

2. Because of the agreement reached with respondents and their employing organizations, pseudonyms will be used when referring to the four hospitals in the study. Furthermore, when quoting or otherwise referring to statements made by interviewees, any reference to the source of such statements will only be in terms of the broad, generic job category occupied by the respondent. Finally, reference is usually made to specialties, not clinical directorates, because there is more inter hospital comparability with respect to the former than the latter.

Acknowledgements

I would like to extend my thanks to the many NHS personnel interviewed. So many people have given generously of their time and, without such support, neither the overall research project nor this part of it would have been possible. However, for reasons made clear in note 2 above, it is not possible to single out any of them for special thanks. However, I can and wish to acknowledge the contribution of David Salt and Juan Baeza, both past research assistants with the NHS Organizational Change Project, for much of the data gathering, and preliminary analysis, on which much of the chapter rests. I also want to thank my wife, Helen Tilley, for her indispensable help as always in the production of this chapter.

References

Appleby, J. (1992), *Financing Health Care in the 1990s*, Open University Press, Buckingham.

Appleby, J. and Little, V. (1993), 'Health and efficiency', *Health Service Journal*, 6 May, pp. 20-22.

Bacharach, S. B. and Lawler, E. J. (1980), *Power and politics in organizations*, Jossey-Bass, San Francisco.

Baeza, J. et al. (1993), 'Four providers' strategic responses and the internal market' in Tilley, Ian (ed.), *Managing the Internal Market*, Paul Chapman, London, pp. 118-137.

Butler, J. (1992), *Patients, Policies and Politics: Before and After 'Working for patients'*, Open University Press, Buckingham.

Butler, P. (1993), 'All change', *Health Service Journal*, 1 July, pp. 10-11.

Crompton, R. and Sanderson, K. (1990), *Gendered Jobs and Social Change*, Unwin Hyman, London.

Department of Health (1990), *National Health Service and Community Care Act*, HMSO, London.

Department of Health (1991), *The Health of the Nation: a Consultative Document for Health in England*, HMSO, London.

Department of Health (1993), *Making London better*, HMSO, London.

Doorslaer, E. K. A. van. and Vliet, R. C. J. A. van. (1989), 'A built bed is a filled bed: an empirical re-examination', *Social Science & Medicine*, pp. 155-164.

Drummond, M. F. et al. (eds), (1993), *Purchasing and Providing Cost-Effective Health Care*, Churchill Livingstone, Edinburgh.

Griffiths, R. (1983), *NHS Management Inquiry Report*, DHSS, London.

Harrison, S. et al. (1992), *Just Managing: Power and Culture in the National Health Service*, Macmillan, London.

Haugaard, M. (1992), *Structures, Restructuration and Social Power*, Avebury, Aldershot.

Johnson, H. T. and Kaplan, R. S. (1987), *Relevance Lost*, Harvard Business School Press, Boston.

Mehafdi, M. (1991), 'A behavioural examination of transfer pricing in large UK firms', unpublished PhD thesis, Business School, University of Greenwich.

Meyer, J. W. and Scott, W. R. (1992), *Organizational Environments: Ritual and Rationality*, updated edition, Sage, Newbury Park, California.

Mintzberg, H. (1983), *Power In and Around Organizations,* Prentice-Hall, Englewood Cliffs, N. J.
NHS (Management) Executive (1991), *The NHS Reforms: the first six months*, HMSO, London.
Pettigrew, A. M. (1975), 'Towards a political theory of organizational intervention', *Human Relations*, pp. 191-208.
Pettigrew, A. M. (1983), 'Patterns of managerial response as organizations move from rich to poor environments', *Educational Management and Administration*, pp. 104-114.
Pettigrew, A. M. (1985), *The Awakening Giant: Continuity and Change in Imperial Chemical Industries*, Blackwell, Oxford.
Pfeffer, J. (1981), *Power in Organizations*, Pitman, Marshfield, Mass.
Rosoff, S. and Leone, M. C. (1991), 'The public prestige of medical specialties: overviews and undercurrents', *Social Science & Medicine*, pp. 321-342.
Salt, D. et al. (1993), 'Researching the Reforms in NHS hospitals', British Academy of Management (BAM) annual conference, Cranfield School of Management/Open University. Business School.
Salt, D. (1994), 'Changes in NHS employment relations: a case study of an NHS hospital', BAM annual conference, Lancaster University.
Smith, P. (1992), *The Emotional Labour of Nursing: How Nurses Care*, Macmillan, London.
Strong, P. and Robinson, J. (1990), *The NHS - Under New Management*, Open University Press, Milton Keynes.
Tilley, I. (ed.), (1993), *Managing the Internal Market*, Paul Chapman, London.
Tilley, I. and Salt, D. (1994), *The Purchasing Process in the Reforming NHS: an explanatory model*, Public Management Paper, Centre for Public Services Management, South Bank University, London.
Tilley, I. et al. (1991), 'Hospital organisation and intra-hospital interest groups', British Sociological Association annual conference, Manchester University.
Tomlinson, B. (1992), *Report of the Inquiry into London's Health Service, Medical Education and Research*, HMSO, London.
Willis, P. E. (1980), *Learning to Labour*, Gower, Aldershot.

8 In or out of management? Dilemmas and developments in public health medicine in England

Sandra Dawson, Jim Sherval and Veronica Mole

Introduction

The reorganization of the National Health Service (NHS) in England into purchasing and providing organizations has changed the role of the District Health Authority (DHA). It has also had an effect on the roles of actors within DHAs. Directors of Public Health (DPHs), and Departments of Public Health in general, have been given an opportunity to exert influence in determining the future shape of health service provision across a wide spectrum of health promotion, illness prevention, treatment and care. The emphasis on improving the health and well being of the population which flows from the reforms accords with the traditional focus and aims of Public Health as a profession. A higher value is now implied for skills that have traditionally been core competences of those located within the Public Health discipline such as epidemiology and health needs assessment.

However, there are many obstacles in the path of those, both within and outside the public health profession, who seek to realise the increased potential for public health to influence purchasing strategy and operations. Three examples illustrate some of the difficulties. Historically, Public Health Physicians (PHPs) have been regarded, within the medical profession, as a group with relatively low status and influence. Yet they are now asked to question more explicitly the efficacy or value of time honoured procedures carried out by established professionals who hitherto have regarded themselves as superior in the 'pecking order' of the medical profession. Secondly, DPHs are required to be part of a strategic managerial process charged with developing a commissioning strategy which will inevitably embody difficult decisions on rationing and priorities, which must be defended and owned as part of corporate managerial responsibility. As DPHs move increasingly to be part of the corporate DHA, their historically established 'independence' will be more difficult to sustain. Finally, as the DHA is now centrally concerned with the pursuit of health gain for its population, questions are asked about the specific contribution of Public Health Medicine.

This chapter draws on a two year project begun in January 1992 and funded by the Department of Health into 'Senior Managerial Competences, Succession Planning and Organizational Development in the NHS'. Fieldwork has been conducted in 10 purchaser and 11 provider organizations. The research team has conducted individual interviews with members of the senior management team in each organization. This chapter draws particularly on interviews with Directors of Public Health and their executive colleagues in 10 DHAs.

The chapter is in three main sections. Section one establishes the context and outlines the changing role of the District Health Authority in the NHS. Section two places the discussion of public health within an historical context. Section three outlines the role of the DPH and addresses some contemporary issues concerning the relationship of the DPH with management through reference to empirical findings.

The context: purchasing for health gain

The recent changes to the health service have been well documented (Ham, 1991; Tilley, 1993). There has been a fundamental redefinition of the role of the District Health Authority. Districts have had a duty to plan and deliver services for their populations for some years since their creation in 1982. However the incentives of the system were such that this objective was not always uppermost in a context which was heavily dominated by an agenda constructed around and by institutional (largely hospital) settings and significant groups of provider professions. In the foreword to the green paper *The health of the nation* the change in the role of DHAs was a 'key feature' in the general thrust of the reforms to the NHS, namely 'to give the Health Service a much greater capacity explicitly to address the health needs of the country.' (Secretary of State 1991, p. iii)

The reforms have concentrated attention away from the funding of institutions to resource allocation based on patient need through the creation of a new environment in which health care is to be delivered. That environment is the internal market in which purchasers (District Health Authorities, General Practitioner Fund Holders) now receive money from the State in proportion to their population figures, weighted for certain indices of disadvantage. Purchasers' remit is to assess local needs and implement the most appropriate ways in which they can be met. They are to consider health promotion and illness prevention as well as the efficacy and value for money of different patterns of care. (Appleby, 1992; Ham, 1991; Harrison, 1988; Mark & Scott, 1992; Strong and Robinson, 1990).

Purchasers have not, however, been given a free hand in deciding the health priorities of their resident populations. They must meet certain national demands and criteria, which act as constraints, or at least strong influences, on the task of purchasing. Central standards need to be successfully married to a vigorous local strategy. Examples of national policies are *The Patients' Charter* (Department of Health, 1992), the waiting list initiative (to reduce waiting times for hospital admissions) and documents on priority and planning guidance from the NHS Executive (eg NHSME, 1992). The espoused aims of improving efficiency, value for money, and effectiveness are threads which run through each initiative. It is expected that corporate contracts and plans between Regional authorities and DHAs will reflect these priorities. It is an irony of the reforms that it is argued that there has been little official guidance on priority setting while at the same time it is plausibly claimed that health authorities are suffering from priority overload (Mooney et al., 1992, Klein and Redmayne, 1992).

Health care has always been rationed. Mechanisms have related to differential ease of access to, or length of wait for, services. Now, however, rationing questions may be debated more openly, because the reforms demand that DHAs develop explicit purchasing plans that focus on areas of priority. The difficulty of finding agreeable ways to assess various interventions and the embryonic nature of purchasing have meant that criteria for purchasing decision making can be more openly contested at least at the margins. However, an analysis of the purchasing plans for 1992-93 concluded that 'the new system has not dented the NHS tradition of almost imperceptible incremental change' (Klein and Redmayne, 1992, p. 23). Money has tended to be spread across priorities with rationing left to the margins with the 'express denial' of some services limited to only 12 health authorities out of the 114 purchasing plans studied (Klein and Redmayne, 1992).

In the first two years of the reforms, until 1993, much governmental, media, academic and service attention had been firmly focused on the development of NHS Trusts as the providers of secondary health care. The spotlight then moved to the huge agenda implied by the need to develop purchasing. This was the subject of a series of ministerial speeches. In the first speech, Dr Mawhinny outlined '7 main stepping stones to effective purchasing' in terms of strategy, effective contracts, knowledge base, responsiveness to local people, mature relations with providers, local alliances, and organizational capacity. Expanding on the last point about organizational capacity, the Minister said that, 'the management and professional expertise of purchasers needs to be strengthened.' (Minister for Health, 1993).

Critical to the delivery of improved purchasing is informed, appropriate and timely advice and information concerning both the needs of the population and the development of services. Public Health Physicians are instrumental in providing this input. The paper now turns to examine how they have reached this position and what, in the present context, facilitates and inhibits their development in what is essentially a managerial role.

Public health: history and tradition

Introduction

This section discusses the historical context of public health. It shows that the recent history of the profession of Public Health has, at a collective level, been one of uncertainty and low morale and status, even though, on an individual level, the picture is often less bleak. The section suggests that while the recent reforms, unlike previous reorganizations, could enhance the position of Public Health, much depends on the individual DPH and his/her relations within purchasing organizations if this potential is to be realised.

Public Health Medicine (PHM) has, like other medical specialties, its own postgraduate training and standards. However, Public Health, perhaps more than any other medical specialty, has had to cope with shifting sands; the basis of its identity and power eroded or redeposited by repeated reorganization and the different preoccupations of more ascendant groups.

Public health has been defined as 'the science and art of preventing disease, prolonging life and promoting health through organised efforts of society' (Acheson, 1988). Perhaps we should speak more of a tradition than a profession as the multi disciplinary nature of public health work is well documented (Alderslade and Hunter, 1992; Thomson and Bhopal, 1993). For over a century and a half medically trained doctors have been working in the generic area which may be called public health, but 'Public Health Medicine' only become the formal professional title of this group in 1988 when it replaced 'Community Medicine'. The direct roots of the profession lie in sanitary reform and the poor laws of the Nineteenth century; the 'pioneers...were all characterised by a social conscience' (John, 1987). Within this tradition, public health is something of a normative profession.

Public health doctors' uncertain relationship with management can be dated to the reorganization of the health service in 1974 when they entered the NHS as a unified group. But their history prior to this is important in terms of the influence it had on subsequent developments.

Pre 1974

Between the wars (1918-1939) Medical Officers of Health (MOHs), working as local authority officers, took on increasing responsibility for the provision of health services in general as well as special responsibility for particular client groups such as children. They sat at the top of a large, hierarchical department with a remit, among other things, to report to the local council on the health of the population. (Lewis, 1987) The MOH could not be dismissed without ministerial consent, a fact which Acheson interpreted as showing that Parliament acknowledged the major importance of public health issues and that 'in discharging duties...the MOH might well fall foul of local vested interests'. Ultimately, without this protection the

MOH 'might be unable to protect the public interest' (Acheson, 1988, p. 91)

The influence of the MOH was at its peak between 1930 and 1948 achieving much integration of what we might term now both health and health care services, that is including both preventative and curative aspects (John, 1987).

The creation of the NHS in 1948 marginalised the MOHs. They were left in local authorities with the remit of coordinating non acute, non general practitioner community services. Bereft of the responsibility for hospitals, which was where the main developments of the service took place in the following decades, the MOHs were increasingly squeezed out of their community role by the developing notion of GP based family health services, and the creation of a separate personal social services department by the Local Authority Social Services Act (1970) (Lewis, 1987).

Post 1974

The 1974 reorganization of the health service attempted to strengthen the service's focus on health rather than just health care, although it is arguable whether this did in fact occur. Acheson (1988) acknowledged the irony that this focus, strong in the 1919 Health act, had been dissipated in the structure chosen in 1948. In parallel to these developments, the faculty of Community Medicine was created in 1972 to bring together all those involved in public health. The creation of the faculty had been recommended by the Hunter Report (1972) as a way of as bringing together three groups; the former MOHs and their staff, the administrative Medical Officers of former hospital boards, and the medical staff of academic departments of public health and social medicine. This has been characterised as the merger of, respectively, disease prevention, medical administration and epidemiology (Thomson and Bhopal, 1993) As the Acheson report (1988) put it 'the 1974 reorganization made possible the recreation of a role lost in 1948 for a single doctor or team of doctors (the Community physicians) to consider and plan for the health needs of the whole population of a district, area or region' (Acheson, 1988, p. 6).

The idea of the community physician had been germinating in public health teaching since the late 50s (Lewis 1987 p. 93), it centred around responsibility for the diagnosis of the health needs of the community, an intelligence function providing information for effective and efficient administration of health services, and generally as a linchpin integrating services that had previously been too divided. However, the delineation of the tasks of the Community physician and particularly the place of management within these tasks was never spelled out. 'As a specialist in population medicine, the Community Physician was intended to be both an advisor to non-medical administrators and clinicians, and a manager with a formal place in the new consensus management structure' (Lewis, 1987, p. 95). The exact balance was left to be worked out on a local basis; this was often done by default reflecting particular individual interests and organizational contexts. The success of Community Medicine came only on an individual level. The specialty as a whole did not establish a status or level of prestige in any way comparable to other medical specialties (Lewis, 1987; John, 1987; Acheson, 1988; Alderslade and Hunter, 1992).

John (1987) feels this failure to fulfil potential was due to over involvement in management with Community Physicians becoming preoccupied with firefighting, mainly financial, crises in the acute sector, and suffering from a simple lack of support staff. Lewis (1987) argues that the lack of operationalization of the position of Community Physician led to it being 'somewhat at the mercy of the new structure'. The Acheson report (1988) agrees that short term pressures eclipsed more strategic views, but also that many Community physicians had a local authority background and could not fully meet the responsibilities of the health authority which included hospitals. Alderslade and Hunter (1992) divide the blame between service managers with their acute-centred concerns and Community Physicians' lack of 'practical and problem solving skills in the management of change'.

The 1980s

Further organizational change in the 1980s did little to boost the position of the Community physicians. The Patients First consultation process (1979-80) resulted in changes to health authorities in 1982. In the same year 20 per cent of the total number of Community physicians took early retirement (Acheson, 1988, p. 7) The NHS Management Inquiry (The Griffiths report) in the next year (1983) added to the decline of the profession's credibility and morale. The implementation of the report allowed authorities much more flexibility in their management arrangements. It was later discovered that 13 authorities had no Community Physician on their management board and many posts still held by Community Physicians had titles such as Director of Planning or Director of Service Evaluation. As such they were, 'describing roles which did not necessarily need a medically qualified specialist to fulfil them' (Acheson, 1988). This further confused the image of public health doctors and exacerbated the spiral of uncertainty in which the profession found itself; poor morale affected the supply and quality of recruits as the number of jobs fell and their nature was unclear.

A survey of public health doctors by Lewis in 1986 and quoted by John (1987) found that they fell into two types. They either saw themselves as medical administrators/ co-ordinators/ firefighters or in more of a strategic function, as radical champions of the public interest. This may in large part account for the confused image of the profession held by many outside it.

The Report of the Committee of Inquiry into the Future Development of the Public Health Function (The Acheson Report, 1988) attempted to affirm the need for doctors in public health in the NHS. The Committee of Inquiry was set up in early 1986 as a direct result of the findings of the public inquiries that followed two separate and major outbreaks of communicable disease. In its terms of reference it was also to consider the effects of the introduction, following Griffiths, of general management into the health service.

In its foreword the report states that:

> The special training of public health doctors in epidemiology - i.e. the study of the distribution and determinants of health and disease in populations - means that they are qualified not only to develop policies for the prevention of illness and promotion of health but, in collaboration with others, to analyse the need for health services and evaluate their outcome. (Acheson, 1988, p. i).

The report went on to define the core tasks of the DPH and colleagues at district level. It noted the implicit nature of the NHS' objective to further health by the prevention of illness and the promotion of healthy lifestyles (Acheson, 1988, p. 14). The report argued that lead responsibility for this objective should be made explicit. Adapting to the introduction of general management following the Griffiths Report, the Acheson Report recommended that the Director of Public Health take up the explicit lead for health promotion and illness prevention and that this position should be held by a consultant in Public Health Medicine. This has been reaffirmed by the Abrams report which added, in the light of the reforms, that the DPH should be an executive member of the DHA (NHSME, 1993).

The Acheson Report also recommended that the DPH should be the chief source of medical advice to the authority and should be a part of the key decision making machinery in the district. There was discussion of the issue of independence but the report rejected the reinstatement of the statutory protection that the MOH had enjoyed and also the idea that being managed by a DPH undermined the status of other consultants in Public Health Medicine in relation to consultants in other medical specialties.

The Acheson Report also made it clear that Public Health doctors 'should frequently act as initiators and catalysts for change'. This suggests that Public Health doctors should be more than simply advisers. Thomson and Bhopal (1993) argue that Public Health doctors can contribute to improvements in the quality of provider based care both indirectly as a purchaser through contracts and directly through collaboration with providers. This view is part of a wider debate about the role and natural home of Public Health Medicine (for example Whitty and Jones, 1992).

The Acheson Report (1988) recommended that the difficulties that the NHS had in addressing issues of the prevention of illness and promotion of health should be tackled by identifying a key player called the Director of Public Health. This was implemented by the circular HC(88)64. However, it could be argued that with the clear delineation of purchasers and providers by the 1991 health reforms, the DHA as a whole is now the key player in addressing the health needs of the population. What then is the specific contribution of Public Health?

Far from consolidating the position of the public health doctor, the reforms, to some extent, have fuelled the debate surrounding the Public Health profession. It has been reported that the number of DPHs and PHPs employed by health authorities is falling because of the mergers of authorities (Health Service Journal, 29 April, 1993, p.16). Also, the title of Director of Public Health has not proved unchangeable with titles such as Director of 'Health Gain', 'Health Strategy' and of 'Health' emerging. This echoes the changes in the names of posts that Community Physicians held after the 1974 reorganization. Two academics, one a senior Public Health doctor have argued for a notion of 'Public Health management' and challenged the idea that the Director of Public Health must be a Consultant in Public Health Medicine, or even a doctor at all, due to the wide variety of professions involved in the delivery of public health tasks (Alderslade and Hunter, 1992).

Thus it can be seen that the Acheson Report's exhortation of the importance of Public Health will not alone preserve the position of the specialty. The roles played by and value placed on the Director of Public Health and their directorate varies widely from purchaser to purchaser. The new commissioning role of districts demands that departmental boundaries become more fluid, and that members of each department or profession should be able to balance on the boundaries integrating contributions from a variety of fields (Dawson, 1993). The Audit Commission (1993, p. 21) mentions the problem of poor integration of the Public Health department into the DHA in some places. This is echoed in the research reported in the next section where complaints about Public Health often suggested that their advice to contract negotiators was impractical. 'Particular directors of public health have had problems reconciling their independent role as guardian of the community's health, with the requirement to participate in such unenviable corporate decisions as deciding which services are affordable' (Audit Commission 1993, p. 25). The Commission advises those responsible for needs assessment to treat contract negotiators as their 'internal customers'.

The internal market may therefore once again have been a reorganization that leaves the profession with an uncertain and contested future.

Directors of public health

Introduction

Data for this chapter is drawn from a wider project on senior executives who were involved in the local purchase or provision of health care in England. Areas of interest were to establish what the executives did, what problems they faced and the extent to which they felt equipped to fulfil the roles and responsibilities demanded of them. Information was also collected on the organizational contexts in which the senior executives worked. Data collection took the form of a personal, semi-structured interview lasting approximately one hour with each participant. It was designed to be administered to every individual respondent taking into account different professional backgrounds and organization types.

This paper draws on answers from 10 of the respondents who were Directors of Public Health. Further contextual information was provided through interviews with four PHPs who were in a Public Health department as consultants, five PHPs who were in other executive or professional advisory posts in DHAs as well as interviews with 85 other senior executives in purchasing organizations, including 34 who, like DPHs, were executive members of DHA boards.

The DPHs interviewed came from five former English regions. One DPH was interviewed in 1992, the remaining 9 were interviewed during 1993. No pretence is made that our group of DPHs is a scientifically established random sample of the national population, however, the geographical and organizational spread does give some basis for generalisability. Interestingly, one generalization that can be made is that anecdotal experience of the practice of Public Health seems to vary so widely in the NHS. There is still sufficient lack of shared agreement nationally about what the role of public health should be, that the performance of the task reflects, perhaps, more than any other function in the DHA, the individual style and preoccupations of the DPH. The findings suggest that the 10 DPHs interviewed are well aware of the management challenge they face. Attitudes to this challenge differ but the extent to which corporate priorities are embraced is high, often resulting in considerable tension to the individual postholder.

Duties and activities of the DPH

Each interviewee was asked to choose from a preselected list of managerial duties and activities and to indicate the degree of importance to them in their job on a scale from little importance to extremely important.

DPHs saw their job as having a core of highly or extremely important managerial activities which were; strategic planning, internal liaison and networking (ie meetings, discussions, communications with other people/professions within the DHA), external liaison and networking (i.e. meetings, discussions, communications with other people/professions and agencies outside the DHA), motivating their team, organising their team, and health needs assessment. The latter can be seen as the inner, professional core of their remit.

This creates a picture in which DPHs see their responsibilities for the internal management of their team as of equal importance to participation in strategic planning and health needs assessment. The legitimacy of having a medical consultant managerially 'in charge' of another is only slowly being acknowledged within the medical profession. In Public Health managerial oversight has been the case for much longer than in clinical medicine; indeed, evidence was given to the Acheson committee which argued that the position of the DPH 'in charge of others' exacerbated the poor image of Public Health held by many doctors. With the rise of clinical directorates in provider units, wherein other doctors as clinical directors now assume managerial responsibility, the DPH no longer looks anomalous within the wider profession.

The respondents also emphasised their role in communication and liaison, not in a hierarchical, managerial mode but in terms of networking and liaison with other groups both internal and external to their organization. The challenge to move away from a hierarchical to a more network based way of working is being experienced across the purchasing sector. It is not just an issue for public health but also for other groups such as finance and quality. The attitudes of the directors involved are crucial to the facilitation of more and better inter-directorate working. The stress on external (to the DHA) liaison and networking reflects the important role the DPH has in the key purchasing task of multi-agency working. It is now acknowledged that Health of the Nation targets cut across health, social services and housing and their pursuit requires effective inter agency working. This was an area in which 9 of the 10 DPH respondents felt they needed significant further management development.

Main barriers

Interviewees were asked what they regarded as the main barriers, if any, that prevented them from doing their job in the way that they would like to do it. Three general themes could be detected from the responses of DPHs. There was a high degree of weariness of organizational change, frustration concerning the availability of information, and cynicism directed towards the centre of the NHS. Each of these barriers represented significant demands on the time which DPHs felt they had to discharge their duties.

Organizational change

All respondents had some comments to make about the constancy of organizational change. Some respondents spoke either about the sheer fact of five reorganizations in ten years, others expressed the view that the purchaser/provider split had in some ways made their job of influencing provision more difficult. This was in part because the created organizational arrangements and, thereby, boundaries, tended to get in the way of providing them with good access to advice and information on services from local providers. It was only a small minority of the 10 who felt that the reforms had empowered them.

Information

All DPH respondents noted significant information barriers including a paucity of cost effectiveness data. They commented on the level of sophistication within Information departments in purchasing as well as in providing and they bemoaned the loss of contact with, or the cageyness of, local clinicians in the provider units. With the lack of good information on some services one DPH felt that the internal market meant he could no longer judge the objectivity of the advice of local clinicians on services as he did not know them so well.

Central control

The third group of 'barriers' concerned the extent of perceived political expediency or short termism which respondents identified as driving forces in the centre of the NHS. This was felt to foster 'a culture of process control' stifling innovation. The requirement to react quickly to the latest promulgated 'flavour of the month' together with the sheer volume of work directed from the centre also gave cause for comment.

Professional-managerial relationships

A theme that recurs in the literature is the uncertain relationship between public health doctors and management. One DPH put a personal view that:

> there is a different value system between managers and Public Health physicians: at its bleakest and briefest Public Health is interested in science and health and getting it right, while managers are interested in pleasing the next layer up and doing it quickly.

Paradoxically, the new opportunities for Public Health embodied in the reforms require those in Public Health to engage directly with management. Their role is to be part of the strategic management of purchasing. A challenge and dilemma for them is to determine the extent to which they can fulfil their strategic roles and yet also retain some spirit of radical independence, that is for those who still feel the latter is an important tradition to maintain.

Even in 1974 some public health doctors saw potential tension between their allegiance to a population and the bureaucracy of the NHS (Lewis, 1987, p. 95). In our study one DPH outlined his career as taking in two views of public health.

The first was the Public Health doctor as 'free radical', a 'gadfly on the side of the organization' asking provocative questions in a sense from the outside. This he felt characterised the earlier part of his career. His second view was that of the 'bureaucratic quisling', swayed by external pressures, with a 'greater consciousness of realpolitik' and aiming for influence from the inside.

There is the possibility that the DPH, due to the influence of tradition and the nature of the Public Health job, may find it difficult to be a 'team player'. Much has already been said about the former independence of the Medical Officer of Health, and also the more normative aspects of the profession. An indication of the extent to which DPHs face this difficulty is found in their replies to a question respondents were asked about the criteria they used to set priorities in their job. Whilst most of them said they took a corporate view on priority setting; they were also strongly oriented towards community objectives. The DPH has editorial independence over the annual Public Health report, and this may be extremely significant in providing an outlet for more individual expression. An independent and individual approach was never far from the surface in the interviews; as one DPH said:

> Many people in Public Health say they are marginalised but this is because they have their own agenda. I spend time getting the district's agenda round to mine.

As regards the relationship between managers and professionals, all respondents were asked whether they thought that people with a clinical or health professional background make a different contribution to the management team than those with a managerial background and if so in what ways.

All 10 DPHs agreed that each group made a different contribution, but views differed in the extent to which they felt that the differences were profound. For some, while they saw public health physicians as professionals bringing a particular knowledge, they felt that much depended on the individual as to what kind of contribution they make. As one DPH put it:

> they are different but its not a problem. The Treasurer (the Finance director) has developed into quite a good amateur Public Health Physician. I have taken on board messages from them (the other directors).

Another DPH said that he had:

> toyed with the idea of becoming ...CEO. I didn't because I very much had the feeling that I wanted to maintain my professional roots and role. I don't have the characteristics to become an apparatchik. If (your boss) says jump you jump as a manager. One is still a corporate beast, in fact you're ineffective if you're just an adviser. But I have another loyalty to the population and patients and (as DPH) I'm able to bring this about.

Another commented:

> I'm definitely the odd one out - as the doctor in the team ... I find compromise difficult.

However, other Public Health doctors are in fact in CEO positions in purchasing agencies and they have felt that there was compatibility and synergy between the two experiences. This lead some to comment on their mediating role. One felt they had:

> ...a facilitative role between purchasers and providers such as to explain that there are such things as cash limits and choices and there's a need for clinicians to get their act together...or else management will do it for them.

In this bridging role one DPH acknowledged that:

> There's some distrust in the doc to doc thing, I'm conscious of a 'where does your heart really lie' challenge ... added to which I can't by myself deliver anything, I can transmit messages and encourage dialogue.

Another commented:

> ... I can do a lot through influence and maintain my professional integrity, we're given real responsibility for patients and politicians ... its right to blow the whistle.

Another DPH outlined a problem with timescales saying that:

> managers go with what they've got on Thursday, whereas professionals will wait until Friday if the information for a better informed decision is only available on Friday.

Seven of the ten DPHs felt that being medically qualified gave them a credibility with providers that managers did not have. In this sense the DPH has a facilitative role in bridging two world views and explaining one to another. As one DPH put it, his professional training as a doctor 'at the sharp end' meant that he knew what it was like to 'have a patient in front of you'. However, he said that he would 'do anything to stop it becoming a them and us situation' by trying to reflect both 'camps' as he felt 'there is appalling ignorance of management and of health by both areas'. To appreciate the difference between two or more contributions does not, of course, involve each becoming identical to the other. Indeed, it can be argued that given the complexity and essentially contested nature of purchasing for health, it is crucial that a variety of perspectives are strongly represented. The

DPH has a particular voice which has been developed through special training and experience. The DPHs encountered in this study were seeking to find ways of making their voice heard so that it is distinctive, yet at the same time central not peripheral. For them the challenging paradox is to be distinct from, and yet part of, the management of purchasing.

Conclusion

We have seen how since 1948 the profession of public health has through various organizational changes found itself somewhat marginalised from the central arena of health provision. Furthermore, it has not been traditionally regarded as a central section of the medical profession. Paradoxically, the NHS reforms provide a sound basis for it to reestablish itself as a key strategic player, but at a possible cost of the loss or compromise of 'independence'. In the present context, its strength and power base is crucially within the purchasing team which has to manage the allocation of scarce resources in order best to meet the needs of local populations.

There is the potential for public health physicians significantly to influence the provision of healthcare and to play a part in securing significant resources for illness prevention and health promotion as well as for cure and treatment. However, the more PHPs take up this challenge, the more they become a part of the managerial tradition. Not only will they be party to decisions to increase investment in certain areas but given the cash limited size of the NHS budget, they will also be party to decisions to decrease and even discontinue investment in others. This means that on the one hand they will not always be able to represent the common man 'from the sidelines' - nor will they always be on the same side of the argument as that adopted by other colleagues in the medical profession.

In our research Directors of Public Health have identified that they face significant internal managerial challenges, to motivate and organise their team and to secure internal communications between different groups within the organization. This however is the more obvious and straightforward part of their managerial agenda. More fundamentally as individuals, and as a professional group, they have to resolve the dilemma of whether they are 'in or out of management' when it comes to managing health care for a local population and, indeed, in managing the market. Perhaps the trick is for them to learn to be both.

References

Acheson Report, Department of Health (1988), *Public Health in England*, HMSO, London.

Alderslade, R. and Hunter, D. (1992), 'Forward March', *Health Service Journal*, 22-23 March.

Appleby, J. (1992), *Financing Health Care in the 1990s*, Open University Press, Milton Keynes.

Audit Commission (1993), *Their Health, Your Business*, HMSO, London.

Dawson, S. (1993), Developing and managing expertise: the challenge for management development, Paper given at the *Institute of Health Service Management* annual conference, 9-11 June, Birmingham.

Department of Health and Social Security (DHSS) (1989), *Working for Patients: the Health Service Caring for the 1990s*, HMSO, London.

Department of Health (1992), *The Patient's Charter: Raising the Standard*, HMSO, London.

Griffiths, R. (1983), *NHS Management Inquiry Report*, DHSS, London.

Ham, C. (1991), *The New NHS Organisation and Management*, Radcliffe Medical Papers, Oxford.

Harrison, S. (1988), *Managing the National Health Service - Shifting the Frontier?* Chapman and Hall, London.

John, H. (1987), 'The Medical Officer of Health: past, present and future' in Farrow, S (ed.), *The Public Health Challenge*, 59-85. Hutchinson, London.

Klein, R. and Redmayne, S. (1992), *Patterns of priorities*, NAHAT research paper 7.

Lewis, J. (1987), 'From public health to community medicine: the wider context' in Farrow, S (ed.), *The Public Health Challenge*, 87-99. Hutchinson, London.

Mark, A. and Scott, H. (1992), 'Management of the National Health Service', in Willcocks, L. & Harrow, J. (eds), *Rediscovering Public Service Management*, McGraw Hill, London.

Minister for Health (1993), *Purchasing for Health: a Framework for Action*, NHSME.

Mooney, G., Gerard, K., Donaldson, C. and Farrar, S. (1992), *Priority Setting in Purchasing*, NAHAT research paper 6.

National Health Service Management Executive (NHSME) (1992), *Priorities and Planning Guidance 1993/94*, EL(92)47.

National Health Service Management Executive (NHSME) (1993), *Public health: Responsibilities of the NHS and the Roles of Others*, HSG(93)56.

Secretary of State for Health (1991), *The Health of the Nation: a Consultative Document for Health in England*, Cm 1523, HMSO, London.

Strong, P. and Robinson, J. (1990) *The NHS under new management*, Open University Press, Milton Keynes.

Thomson, R. and Bhopal, R. (1993), 'Improving quality of health care: the role of public health medicine' *Quality in Health Care* 2: 35-39.

Tilley, I. (ed.), (1993), *Managing the Internal Market*, Paul Chapman, London.

Whitty. P, and Jones. I (1992), 'Public health heresy: a challenge to the purchasing orthodoxy', *British Medical Journal,* 304: 1039-1041.

9 Doctors in management: A challenge to established debates

Sue Dopson

Introduction

Academics have been fascinated by the medical profession. Doctors and medical power have been the subject of a weighty literature spanning the sociology of the professions, medical sociology, health care management and organizational behaviour. However, most of the debate has been at a conceptual level, for example, examining the nature of doctors' power, the relationship between the profession and the State as well as the difference between professional work and bureaucracy. Relatively little work has been done exploring the doctors' role in the management of health services and even less work has been done exploring the implications of recent moves to involve doctors more closely in the management process.

This chapter considers what we do know about doctors' involvement in the management of health services, drawing on the available ethnographies of health care management. This serves as a backdrop for consideration of the experience of a small sample of consultants moving into clinical director roles or equivalent. Specifically, the chapter considers the extent to which this group of consultants feel consultants' roles have changed, in what ways they have changed and, the concerns they have about the involvement of doctors in management. Finally, the chapter ends with a plea for more research that acknowledges the complexity of the issues surrounding the involvement of doctors in management.

Doctors' involvement in management: The evidence

Perhaps the first question to ask is why successive governments since 1970 have sought to involve doctors more closely in the management of the NHS. In general, the views of consumers and the providers of NHS services - although far from systematically documented - appear to reflect a positive acceptance of the NHS, and a feeling that, although efforts should be made to improve it, there should be no question of dismantling or radically changing it, or that doctors' involvement in the NHS should be significantly altered. There were, however, a number of concerns about the way in which health services were developing in the early 1970s. Firstly health care costs were escalating. The UK in 1969 spent 6 per cent of GNP on health, compared to 3.5 per cent in 1950. Increased costs were related to more advanced medical technology, increased capacity to cure or curtail previously life-threatening diseases, and increased demands for more long-term rehabilitation care. A second concern was the changing population structure and patterns of illness. As acute conditions were prevented or in some cases cured, the population aged and, as a result, the NHS has to cope with more chronic illness which added to the escalating costs. Thirdly, there seemed to be significant local and regional inequalities in terms of allocation of funds to different parts of the country. The DHSS figures at the time suggested that the single most important factor in explaining the allocation of funds in this period, was the historical legacy of each region. Fourthly, a number of scandals during the 1960s, prominent amongst them the Ely mental hospital scandal, served to alert the public to the problems of what were to become known as the 'cinderella services' (mental health, geriatrics and community care services), as well as poor links between hospital and community sectors which threatened 'comprehensive care'. It was as a consequence of these pressures that the power of doctors to shape patterns of care and add significantly to health care costs was questioned in a more rigorous fashion.

The 1974 reorganization of the NHS was the first significant attempt to manage clinician power. The reorganization gave representatives of doctors an important role in the management of health services. A consultant and GP representative, along with an administrator, nurse, treasurer and medical officer, worked as a consensus management team charged with managing health services. The various ethnographic studies carried out of local health care systems constitute an important source of information with which to examine the assumption that consensus management and an essentially bureaucratic reorganization were the way to deal with clinician influence on health services. Stephen Harrison has provided a useful summary of this research between 1948 and 1983 (Harrison, 1988, Chapter 3). In terms of doctors' involvement in the management of health services, ethnographers of local health systems have noted a marked contrast between doctors' involvement on the national and local stage. Nationally doctors have taken a lead in securing a position of influence in both the formation of the NHS and subsequent reorganizations in 1974 and 1982 (Eckstein, 1958; Forsyth, 1966; Haywood and

Alaszewski; 1980).   However, on the local stage, there appears to be a great reluctance on the part of doctors to get involved in local management of health services. Representatives of the profession are shown to be unwilling to give the time to the demands of representative role (Brown, 1979, p.140) and feel vulnerable when taking decisions because of the lack of information and for fear of offending their colleagues (Schultz and Harrison, 1983, p. 29).   In part, the reluctance to be involved in managing local health care delivery can be explained by the over-complicated medical advisory machinery created in 1974, but the most significant reason suggested by available studies is that doctors have a great influence on the patterns and priorities of health care without needing to take up formally-defined administrative roles. Ham succinctly summarises the majority of the available studies when, drawing on the findings of Alford's work (Alford, 1975) he notes:

> The history of hospital planning between 1948 and 1974 can be seen as the history of corporate rationalizers represented by Regional Board planners, trying to challenge the established interests of the medical profession with the community hardly in ear-shot. (Ham, 1981, p. 75)

The available ethnographies of local health service management consistently question the assumption of both the 1974 and 1982 restructurings that management is a rational process where policy is made by the Centre, transmitted to the periphery and implemented there. Health care systems can, and do, circumvent national policies. Studies reveal that decisions affecting local health care delivery evolve in bargaining situations. However, although policy processes at a local level are incremental and plural, the distribution of power is weighted towards the medical profession. Interestingly, the findings of the existing empirical studies of local health care systems did not inform the third reorganization of the NHS which followed the publication of the Griffiths Report in 1983. This reorganization dispensed with the system of consensus management and replaced it with a general manager from any discipline. Griffiths saw general managers as the lynch-pin of dynamic management. They were cast as chief executives, providing leadership and capitalizing on existing high levels of dedication and expertise among NHS staff of all disciplines. In addition, general managers were expected to stimulate 'initiative, urgency and vitality' amongst staff, to bring about a constant search for major change in cost improvement, to motivate staff and ensure that professional functions were effectively fed into the general management process.

Implicit in the Report are two important assumptions with respect to doctors. Firstly, that the development of budgets at unit level would lead to closer involvement of clinicians in managing resources and allow workload service objectives to be related to financial and manpower allocations. Secondly, that members of the medical profession would become general managers. Additionally, other Griffiths recommendations such as the need to ensure that the NHS has a performance orientation as well as a consumer orientation, clearly reinforces the message that the power of the professions, particularly the medical profession, needed to be curtailed. The Griffiths Report represented a distinctly different approach to managing medical power and reflects a more critical attitude towards the power of doctors to shape patterns of care and their dominant position in the doctor-patient relationship. This more aggressive stance by the government was fuelled by many complex factors (for a useful discussion of these see Harrison, 1988, Chapter 6), most prominent of which was the need to rein-in public expenditure.

In practice, only a few general managers came from a medical background and there has been a subsequent decline in numbers (Mark, 1991, p. 6) and management budgeting has met with variable results (Harrison, Hunter, Marnoch and Pollitt, 1989). In short, the consensus of the available commentaries on general management in the NHS[1] has been that the cultural change from the administration of health services to the management of health services with professionals playing a key role has been slow to emerge. More specifically, general managers have been singularly unsuccessful in involving clinicians in managing their services, in changing the pattern of health services and enhancing consumer power. As Harrison notes:

The prime determinant of the pattern of services is still just as before Griffiths, what doctors choose to do. (Harrison, 1988, p. 123).

Exploring the reluctance of doctors to be involved in management

Although many empirical studies have highlighted the reluctance of doctors to be involved in management as a key issue in health care management, very little progress has been made in understanding the problem (Harrison et al., 1993). There are a number of explanations offered. Most frequently cited explanations centre on the power of doctors (often linked to the claim of clinical autonomy) to influence patterns and priorities of health care and the view that bureaucracy and professional work are incompatible (Scott, 1966; Davies, 1983).

The power of hospital clinicians to shape health services has been attributed to many factors including: the concessions made to the doctors in 1948 (Willcocks, 1967; Eckstein, 1958 and 1960); the spread of the epidemic iatrogenesis which has cost humanity its liberty with regard to our own bodies (Illich, 1975), the role of doctors as the agents of capitalism, benefitting from a capitalist system (Navarro, 1978 and 1980); and the objectification of the body (Foucault, 1973). The origin of medical power can, however, be traced back much further. Waddington (1984) notes the importance of the 1858 Medical Act and of the formalization of codes of medical ethics in facilitating the development of a single, relatively unified profession, thus enhancing the power of all medical practitioners. Such explanations have not in themselves proved helpful in either understanding the relationship between doctors and managers or understanding the reluctance of profession, thus enhancing the power of all medical practitioners. Such explanations have not in themselves proved helpful in either understanding the relationship between doctors and managers or understanding the reluctance of doctors to become involved in management. The reality is that doctors and managers have very different interests and perspectives which make the establishment of harmonious relations difficult to achieve. One way of analysing these differences is in terms of Fleck's concept of thought style (Fleck, 1979). Fleck argues that any kind of cognition is a social process. Truth is neither relative and subjective nor absolute and objective, but essentially determined and measured by a given thought style (*Denkstil*). A thought style functions by constraining, inhibiting and determining the way of thinking of individuals. Under the influence of a thought style, one cannot think in any other way, for it excludes alternative modes of perception. Accordingly, no proper communication can arise between those who exhibit different thought styles. A thought style functions at such a fundamental level that the individual is generally unaware of it and its constraining character.

Fleck notes that thought collectives are communal carriers of a given thought style. He defines the thought collective as 'a community of persons mutually exchanging ideas or maintaining intellectual interaction' (Fleck, 1979, p.38). What links the individuals of a thought collective together is the thought style they share. Considered in its collective function, a thought style is a 'special carrier for the historical development of any field of thought, as well as for the given stock of knowledge and level of culture' (Fleck, 1979, p. 39). Doctors and managers have very different 'thought styles' arising from membership of different 'thought collectives'. General Managers tend to stress the virtues of interpersonal skills and of enlisting the cooperation of others. They expect to subsume individual interests to those of the organization. They are also trained to be aware of the wider implications of any activity within the organization. They expect to make optimal use of limited resources and are used to working towards long-term goals. Doctors, in contrast, are expected to strive for the best available evidence before making a decision. They are used to working to short-term operational goals. Furthermore, doctors are hardened by a career-progression which makes tough physical and emotional demands on them and tends to limit their social contacts to people working in the hospital. They rarely receive any training in management or organizational skills until they are quite senior. There is therefore a fundamental conflict of interests on a social structural level, yet often government, general managers, doctors and health service commentators seem to regard the conflict between doctors and managers as simply a conflict on the level of ideas about the relative merits or demerits of management. Furthermore, managers tend to resort to conventional management ideology in dealing with these differences, for example, arguing for change in management strategies.

Recent developments

Since the publication of the 1989 White Paper outlining the latest reorganization of the NHS based on an internal market model, there has been a significant increase in the activity targeted towards involving doctors in management. Ham and Hunter have helpfully outlined three strategies for managing clinical activity following the White Paper changes. They are arranged along a continuum of minimal to maximal involvement by external agents.

(a)	Raising Professional Standards	*Medical Audit *Standards and Guidelines *Accreditation
(b)	Involving Doctors in Management	*Budgets for Doctors *Resource Management Initiative *Doctor-Managers
(c)	External Management Controls of Doctors	*Managing Medical Work *Changing Doctors' Contracts *Extending Provider Competition

Figure 9.1   Strategies for managing clinical activity

Source: *Ham, C. and Hunter, D.J. Managing Clinical Activity in the NHS*, Briefing Paper 8. Kings Fund Institute London 1988. (Cited in Hunter, 1991 p. 444)

The first strategy focuses on encouraging self-help in doctors to raise professional standards by medical audit and the use of standards and guidelines. The second, relies on involving doctors in management by delegating budgetary responsibility to doctors and appointing doctors as managers. The final strategy rests on an attempt to buttress external management control by changing doctors' contracts and encouraging managers to supervise medical work more closely.

Policy makers and senior management in the NHS have concentrated on the second of these strategies in their efforts to manage clinical activity. For example: the resource management initiative (which replaced early experiments of management budgeting, but which is similarly intended to bring doctors into management), has been rolled out of the 12 hospitals and community pilot sites to traditional sites (Hunter, 1991, p. 443); in most hospitals in the NHS, clinical directorates have been set up to manage a budget, although they have considerable responsibilities covering issues such as outpatient scheduling, inpatient admissions, quality assurance, customer relations and medical nursing resources and consultants have been encouraged to take on the job of clinical director or equivalent, responsible for activities in the clinical directorate and supported by a business-manager and a nurse-manager. The rest of this article considers the issues surrounding the movement of hospital consultants into management roles - the doctor-manager option in Hunter's terms.

The doctor-manager

The opportunity to explore the movement of hospital consultants into management roles came via my role as course director for a general management programme for hospital consultants from the Oxford Region. The funding for this programme came from a successful bid to the Department of Health's 'Business School Management Training for Consultants Initiative'. Although the guidance for this initiative originally envisaged that regions would send their doctors on established senior management courses for executives from the private sector, Oxford put forward a different design. It was felt that key clinicians would find it very difficult to leave their work for 4 to 5 consecutive weeks (the average length of such programmes). Sixteen consultants across the region were recruited by the regional training department and the programme began in September 1990. It consisted of four modules of three days each: managing the job/people management; managing finance and information; business planning/strategy and managing key relationships. The course was subject to a local evaluation organized by Oxford Region and Templeton College and to a national evaluation undertaken by the Department of Management Learning, Lancaster University and Middlesex University. It has now been run three times. Funding for the last two groups has come mostly from the Region with some provider contribution. As part of the local evaluation process participants were interviewed, not only about what they found most useful about the programme and what difference, if any, it had made to how they approached their jobs, but the interview explored the changing patterns of their involvement in management over time, the concerns they had about being in management and their management development needs.

Each consultant participating on the first two programmes was interviewed using a semi-structured interview schedule for between an hour and two hours. Those participating on the first course were interviewed twice, towards the end of their course and a year afterwards. I also observed all the teaching sessions on the course and was able to see at first hand, reactions from the participants to the various ideas and frameworks discussed. I also had a great deal of informal contact and discussion in between sessions. This was a very rare and much appreciated opportunity since various researchers have documented how difficult it is to get hospital consultants to give up the time to be interviewed or to become involved in any social science research. (Brazell, 1987). The sample characteristics are given in Table 9.1.

Table 9.1
Characteristics of consultants interviewed

SPECIALTY	CONSULTANT NUMBERS
Anaesthetics	4
Psychiatry	4
Haematology	1
Radiology	1
Physician	3
Pathology	2
Surgery	4
Obstetrics & Gynaecology	3
Paediatrics	3
Plastic Surgery	1
Genetics	1
ENT	1
Oncology	1
Rheumatology	2
Genito-Urinary Medicine	1
Total	32

Such a small scale study cannot do anything but give a flavour of the issues surrounding the movement of hospital consultants into management roles. Furthermore it is a very atypical sample in that doctors have shown an interest in management and have been willing to give time to exploring management issues in a business school environment. Nonetheless, it is offered as a contribution to a debate not known for being grounded in empirical work (Hadley and Foster, 1993, p. 2).

Has professional work changed?

The majority of the consultants interviewed confirmed the findings of the ethnographies of local health management, that the introduction of general management had not made a significant difference to the doctors' role, their involvement and understanding of management, nor, in their view, had general management significantly improved patient care. However, most acknowledged that the introduction of the internal market had resulted in significant change for those consultants who had taken on the role of clinical director or equivalent. This group were reported as having significant responsibility for budgets, strategy and people. Interestingly their job-descriptions did not reflect what they felt was the core of the job, that of influencing their colleagues to think about the future development of the service in the context of limited resources and in a competitive environment. FitzGerald has also noted that although clinical managers often define their own roles in terms of high levels of change management, the job descriptions of clinical directors in her sample focused on the conventional managerial tasks of staff management, team management; representation; and setting and monitoring performance standards (FitzGerald, 1995). It appears from FitzGerald's work and the findings from this sample that the clinical directors' roles have been modelled on an average general management role, instead of seeing them as a unique role.

 All the sample argued that there had been an increase in the interest of their colleagues in management and in the structures within which they now worked, but only in the sense of understanding how management processes and structures would affect how they worked. Most interviewees were quick to point to the existence of a strong powerful group of die-hards who 'hold the view that the NHS should provide all the resources they require'. Several commented on the existence of two polar opposite groups of doctors: one group who 'bury themselves in a hole and look after patients and they pop up every now and then and say how bloody awful it is and then disappear again', and the other group who recognize the need to look at 'the totality of patient care and make sure the facilities are good and that what you are trying to achieve is on a hospital-wide basis'. A few interviewees noted that the lack of interest in management by large sections of the consultant population was hardly surprising given the 'patchy' nature of the market. For example, one member of the sample argued:

 What consultants hear is that things are changing, but what they experience is that things are the same. After an initial flurry of service agreements, negotiations and producing information with purchasers, what has happened in many places is business as usual in the sense of bailing out people who had overspent, agreements being abandoned half way through the year. The system is there in name, but in fact the same people are still operating in the same way.

Why do consultants get involved in management?

Interviewees mentioned several factors aside from the purchaser/provider shake-up, which they felt had facilitated the involvement of consultants in management. The most frequently mentioned reason was the fear consultants had of being managed. As one put it: 'I am not having somebody who isn't a consultant telling me what to do about my service'. Most consultants interviewed were well aware that if they did not take on a management role, then somebody else would do it for them and this was not necessarily in their or their services best interest. The second most frequently given reason for their involvement was concern about the quality of NHS management. Many felt that consultants could not do a worse job managing the NHS than managers had already done. About a quarter of the sample admitted they took up the role because they were bored.

> One of the drawbacks of being a consultant is that you get the job and that is it for 25 years. Faced with this, management becomes an attractive option.

A few were up front about the fact that they saw involvement in management as increasing their power-base. This group firmly believed that doctors get involved in management for professional protection, to protect their department and to ensure they know what is going on. The one consultant who completed her time as clinical director during the course said that 'management is a difficult thing to give up. I am aware things aren't routed to me any more and I miss not knowing what is going on'. One interviewee said he found management intensely exciting and this was what kept him in the role: 'It is a wonderful feeling you get from turning a committee round. It is really sexy.' Only six of the sample said they had taken up the role because of a genuine interest in seeing how management could improve their service. However, this more 'positive' reason has to be balanced by the fact that the majority of interviewees were reluctant to enter management, did so for one or more of the reasons discussed above, or were bullied into it, or it was a case of 'muggin's turn'. All participants predicted a surge of interest in management when consultants realize that their jobs may be at risk.

Concerns about consultant involvement in management

Four major concerns were given by all sample members. Firstly the failure of the government to face up to what the involvement of doctors in management means in resource terms. Several interviewees saw the government's reluctance to properly fund clinical management posts as evidence of government's ambivalence to the idea. Most sample members had been given a session[2] in which to do their management work, which they considered a joke, insulting and yet another indication of how government despised them and the NHS. A second concern centred on a fear of alienating colleagues and undermining clinical relationships. Many interviewees spoke of their involvement in management jeopardising previously good relationships with medical colleagues. At least three of the sample said that a three year reign as clinical director did not offer enough security to take the necessary risks that might influence professional colleagues behaviour in any significant way.

The third major concern given by all the sample was the impact of management work on clinical work. Giving time to management work meant in practice less time for research, teaching and keeping up with developments in their own speciality. The penalties for spending less time on clinical work were obvious to most of the interviewees, the benefits of spending time on management were distinctly hazy. The lack of obvious benefits, coupled with the absence of a real career path for doctors going into management meant that they deliberately limited the time and effort spent engaging in work they termed managing.

The resources given to health care was given as a fourth major concern. As one consultant put it:

> The majority of consultants view the NHS as under-resourced and under-valued by the present political masters, therefore feel it is not a good time to get involved in management....Management is currently seen as having to live within resources that are totally inadequate for health needs.

A number of other concerns were mentioned. Several interviewees noted that time spent on management meant 'dumping clinical work on overworked colleagues'. Most interviewees felt guilty about 'dumping' as they did about being involved in decisions that would affect colleagues. For example:

> If your hospital is vulnerable in a contracting process, you might end up with the distasteful task of overseeing the demise of colleagues and departments because the work isn't coming in.

Inadequate support for their management work was frequently mentioned as a concern. In particular, the absence of sensible secretarial and administration support, poor information and the conventional hours worked by managerial colleagues.

> Management tend to work 9.00 - 5.00. Management people aren't around when I do my management work, i.e. early in the morning or evening.

The attitudes of other health workers were thought by some interviewees to be hindering both the enthusiasm of consultants to become involved in management and their ability to manage effectively. Chief executives were singled out by half the sample as being unhelpful, mainly because they were thought not to want to let go of power. The doctor-bashing attitudes of other professional groups were also commented on.

The low status of management in the NHS was given as yet another factor inhibiting doctors' involvement in management. As one consultant noted:

> The prevalent attitude amongst consultants is that any fool can do management. They think it is all commonsense. They think it is easy compared to the serious business of medicine.

Less frequently mentioned were the following concerns about the involvement of doctors in management. These included: loss of income private practice, the harmful negative attitudes of the BMA and the loneliness of the role 'consultants rarely talk to each other about clinical matters, let alone management'.

It was noted by approximately three-quarters of the sample that the NHS had done quite well with doctors being doctors. Some strongly felt that managers and the government in particular were passing the buck, saying 'it's all your responsibility, it is all your fault the NHS is in the mess it is', without actually giving doctors the resources and the skills that they need to cope with having both a management and clinical role. Interesting, not having management skills was either not mentioned by members of the sample or occasionally referred to. One consultant went so far as to say: 'I have a real fear of realizing that management is difficult.'

Discussion

The feeling amongst this sample of consultants was that the government ought to be facing up to the ethical and value for money issues raised by nudging (in most cases shoving) consultants into what are at present temporary management roles. Many of this sample struggled themselves and with each other, to answer a number of tough, emotionally laden questions. For example: Is my involvement in management actually benefitting patients? Is taking on a management role worth the aggravation with colleagues and worth the increased time and effort put into my work life at the expense of home life? Time devoted to management is time away from patients and research that might benefit patient care, is this ethical? Why spend x thousands of pounds on my management development needs when there are managers in the NHS whom I could advise?

Consultants in this sample often felt guilty about the money spent on their management development, particularly when there is no obvious career path for them to follow. They then were furious that after the investment made in them, they were left on their own again, without any further management development. Most interviewees felt that if the government was serious about making doctors aware of the importance of managing scarce resources, then management development ought to be provided much earlier in the doctors' career, although there was some debate as to when this should be. Some participants felt management skills, especially communication and presentation skills, should be part of the undergraduate programme. Others believed it was too early and would be a wasted input because management seems so far off at that stage and undergraduates might be switched off. Most interviewees favoured management development being targeted at senior registrar level, (the post prior to becoming a consultant) partly because 'it is only then that doctors know where their careers are likely to end up' and partly because senior registrars 'would see the value of acquiring management skills which they could put into practice quite soon'.

The management development programme at Oxford has given participants they say, 'some tools to assist them in the management aspect of their job'. For example, participants argue they can probably better negotiate, manage budgets, ask relevant questions about strategy and manage their time better. The course has been successful in demystifying some of the management jargon they hear so much of. The most frequently mentioned benefit of the course, however, has been the confidence they have gained and the reassurance that what they were doing could be termed management and that other colleagues found it difficult. (Interestingly the willingness of course members to share personal experiences has decreased as time has gone on reflecting the fact that they are now in a more competitive situation). However, the research findings reported here demonstrate that most consultants are reluctant managers. As one consultant put it: 'management is the one disease I did not think existed'.

It is not only the government that ought to be addressing what increasing the involvement of doctors in management actually means in practice. The Royal Colleges, Medical Schools and the BMA have to take seriously the implications of doctors' increased role in management when considering what is appropriate medical education for doctors in the 1990s and beyond as well as the implications of increasing management responsibilities for doctors' careers. The existence of doctors who actively manage their service, their colleagues and the previously untouchable concept of clinical autonomy, also challenge academics to come up with new ideas and new models of professional work.

The literature that explores the relationships between doctors and managers at a local level suffers because it fails to locate empirical work in a convincing theoretical framework. Often the literature discusses these relationships in terms of face-to-face relationships, i.e. how doctors and managers relate to one another, rather than seeing them as part of complex social relationships involving differing power relationships. Doctors and managers are influenced by people and groups they have never seen: government, the press, the Management Executive, for example, are key players. The tendency for researchers to think of relationships in largely individualistic terms reflects the fact that in the course of development of most western societies people have come to experience themselves increasingly strongly as separate beings - district both from other people and from natural objects and the fact that professional work has not of late been the subject of serious and consistent attention.

Future debates on the involvement of doctors in management not only need to acknowledge the problems associated with modelling the clinical director post on an average general manager role, but also need to recognise the conflict of interests that exist on a social-structural level between doctors and managers. Furthermore frameworks need to incorporate human emotions and conceptualise human beings as they really are, involved emotional beings. Questions doctors asked in my sample, about the implications of being involved in management were emotional ones, for example: 'What does the change mean for me?'; 'What are the implications of the change in terms of how my work is being valued?'; 'Is my work being demoted?'; 'Does this mean people don't value me, don't value my work?'; 'What are the implications for my sense of self-worth?'. In speaking negatively about management the sample doctors were not just defending occupational interests on a rational level, but were, in part, defending their self-image as a person doing a good and worthwhile job that is being threatened by other people who do not understand, for example, the nature of clinical medicine. What researchers have to confront is that there are different people/groups within the NHS who perceive their, and other people's interests with varying degrees of accuracy. There are different groups able to act with different balances of emotive and cognitive intellectual processes and are able, with differing degrees, to distance distance themselves and stand back with a degree of detachment and different groups who have differential access to information. Within a complex organizational structure like the NHS, there are a multiplicity of groups, some acting in a more rational, some in a less rational way, or a more involved or less involved way, some groups with more access to information which will aid their decision-making, other groups with less access to the information they need in order to take rational decisions. There is also a variety of groups with different career interests and these are emotive as well as cognitive, who will be struggling over those. Unless more empirical work is done looking at the complexity of the issues surrounding doctors moving into management roles, then the debate is unlikely to get beyond definition mongering.

Notes

1. These ethnographies are reviewed in Harrison, S., Hunter, D., Marnoch, G. and Pollitt, C. (1993), *Just Managing: Power and Culture in the National Health Service*, Macmillan Press.
2. A session is the equivalent of four hours work. This means either the consultant gets paid for an extra session, or he/she is given four hours reprieve from consultant work.

References

Alford, R. R. (1975), *Health Care Politics*, Chicago Ill., University of Chicago Press.

Brazell, H. (1987), 'Doctors as Managers', *Management Education and Development*, 81(2): 95-102.

Brown, R.G.S. (1979), *Reorganizing the National Health Service: A Case Study of Administrative Change* Oxford: Blackwell & Martin Robertson.

Davies, C. (1983), 'Professional in Bureaucracies: The Conflict Thesis Revisited', in Dingwall, R. and Lewis, P. (eds), *The Sociology of Professions*, Macmillan Press.

Eckstein, H. (1958), *English Health Service*, Harvard University Press.

Eckstein, H. (1960), *Pressure Group Politics,* Allen and Unwin.

Fleck, L. (1979), 'Genesis and Development of a Scientific Fact', in Robert K. Merton (ed.), *Genesis and Development of a Scientific Fact*, University of Chicago Press.

FitzGerald, L. (1995), 'Clinical Management: The impact of a changing context on a changing profession', in Leopold, J. W., Glover, I. A. and Hughes, M. D. (eds), *Beyond Reason?*, Avebury, Aldershot.

Forsyth, G. (1966), *Doctors and State Medicine: A study of the British National Health Service*, London: Pitman Medical.

Foucault, M. (1973), *The Birth of the Clinic,* Tavistock, London.

Griffiths, R. (1983), *DHSS, NHS, Management Inquiry*, London: DHSS.

Hadley, R. & Foster, D. (eds), (1993), *Doctors as Managers Experiences in the Front-line of the NHS*, Longman.

Ham, C.J. (1988), *Policy Making in the National Health Service*, London: MacMillan.

Ham, C. and Hunter, D. J. (1988), *Managing Clinical Activity in the NHS,* Briefing Paper 8, Kings Fund Institute, London.

Harrison, S. (1988), *Managing the National Health Service: Shifting the Frontier?*, London, Chapman and Hall.

Harrison, S. (1989), *General Management in the NHS: before and after the White Paper*, Leeds, Nuffield Institute.

Harrison, S., Hunter D., Marnoch, G. & Pollitt, H.C. (1993), *Just Managing: Power and Culture in the National Health Service*, Macmillan Press.

Haywood, S., Alaszewski, A. (1980), *Crisis in the NHS.* London: Croom Helm.

Hunter, D.J. (1991), 'Managing Medicine: A Response to the Crisis', *Social Science and Medicine, Vol.32, no.4, pp.444-49.*

Illich, I. (1975), *Limits to Medicine*, Marion Boyars, London.

Mark, A. (1991), 'Where are the Medical Managers?', *Journal of Management in Medicine*, vol. 5, no. 4, pp. 6-12.

Navarro, V. (1978), *Class Struggle: The State and Medicine*, Martin Robertson, Oxford.

Navarro, V. (1980), 'Work Ideology and Science: The Case of Medicine', *Social Science and Medincine*, Vol. 14, pp. 191-205.

Schultz, R.I. & Harrison, S. (1983), *Teams and Top Managers in the NHS: A Survey and a Strategy*, London: Kings Fund Project Paper, No.41.

Scott, W.R. (1966), 'Professionals in Bureaucracies: Areas of Conflict'. In H.

Vollmer & D. Mills (eds), *Professionalisation*, Englewood Cliffs: N. J., Prentice Hall.

Waddington, I. (1984), *The Medical Profession in the Industrial Revolution*, Gill and Macmillan.

Willcocks, A. J. (1967), *The Creation of the National Health Service,* Routledge and Kegan Paul, London.

10 Clinical management: the impact of a changing context in a changing profession

Louise FitzGerald

Introduction

From political, social and economic perspectives, the position of 'professional' groups within today's society is under debate. Arguments abound that the post-industrial or post-modern society will be increasingly dependent on 'knowledge' workers for competitive advantage, through innovation. (Bell, 1973; Zuboff, 1988; Prahalad and Hamel, 1990; Senge, 1991). Meanwhile, there are many political pressures to curb the power of 'professional' groups. Alongside these pressures, there is an explosive increase in newer bodies of knowledge with their own 'specialists' and 'experts'. These developments raise questions about the continuing utility of the term 'professional' in the world of today. Historically, the specialist expertise of doctors and their collective position as a profession has led to them establishing a position as an exemplar 'profession'. Currently, the adoption of management roles by clinicians is a useful vehicle for the discussion of some of the wider issues, relating to changes in professions and professional power.

This chapter primarily draws on the results of a recently completed research project which tracks a cohort of clinicians as they assume management responsibilities and follows their progress as they undertake training at business schools. (FitzGerald, 1993). However, these data will be complemented by the results from a larger project focussing on the operation of the 'new' boards of the District Health Authorities (DHAs), Trusts and Family Health Services Authorities (FHSAs). This latter study examines clinicians as they operate in a mixed group with managers, dealing with largely non-clinical issues. (See for example, Ashburner, Ferlie and Fitzgerald, 1993).

The methodology adopted in both research projects is a longitudinal one. The primary project collected data in stages examining processes over time. This enabled the clinician's situation prior to training to be examined, and data to be gathered at a number of key stages, during and after the training period. In order to understand the professional position of the clinician, one must analyse the context in which he/she works. This approach of contextualising the doctors' position is a key feature of this analysis. Previous research has been criticised for failing to take account of the socio-political context in which the profession is currently operating (Davies, 1983).

All professional groups are undergoing continuing changes in the boundaries of their professional arenas and are subject to the dynamics of the socio-political context, which influences the value placed on their work. Thus using a methodology which embeds the individual in a context and traces that context longitudinally through time is a route to understanding the changing nature of professions. In this study, it was also important to adopt a methodology that produced an account of development and progression through time, in a context which is changing rapidly. Whilst the data are insufficient to track trends, they do offer indicators of the direction and implications of change.

The characteristics of the cohort are also pertinent. The cohort is small and consists of thirty one clinicians who were assuming or had assumed management roles, mainly as Clinical Directors or as Medical Directors within a healthcare provider unit. All of these roles carry major management responsibilities; but the role of Medical Director would usually be the most senior and carry automatic membership of the Board. As one example of the level of management responsibility, by the latter phases of the study, virtually all clinical managers were budget holders with budgetary responsibility ranging from £4.5 million to £1.9 million. Medical Directors had corporate budgets ranging from £36 to £42 million. The clinicians in the cohort come from a wide range of specialisms; both acute medicine e.g. anaesthetics, surgery, or obstetrics and gynaecology, as well as community health and psychiatry. The doctors are in the age range 35-56, with an average age of 44. Within the group, there are twenty six males and five females.

Using the research data, a number of core themes will be addressed in the chapter. The first theme examines the way the changes in the current context of the healthcare system in the U.K. impact on individual clinicians. The second theme focusses on the impact of these changes, particularly the introduction of a quasi-market in health care, on the intra professional boundaries and on the interfaces between doctors and managers.

Throughout, in discussing the results from the projects, these will be related to a number of the debates raised in the literature. Much discussion has focussed on whether the medical profession, particularly in the U.S.A. can be said to have and be maintaining a position of dominance. Freidson (1984, 1986, 1987) argues cogently that the medical profession has maintained it's dominance through a process of adaptation. He and other writers (McKinlay, 1988) acknowledge the threats that are apparent in the current situation and the major transformation of healthcare systems in developed countries. Nevertheless, Freidson argues that the medical profession has retained control and influence over key areas. Hafferty's (1988) work sets out the threats to the dominance of the medical profession within the current context. This list provides a useful starting point for examining specific issues in the light of the changes under examination. He suggests five areas of threat, which are :

A marketplace in healthcare increases competition between professionals and causes divisions.

Rifts develop within the profession between the clinical managers and the clinicians who are being managed.

External control directly or indirectly limits and reduces the autonomy of the profession eg via General Management in the U.K. or through Administrators and protocols in the USA.

Consumer knowledge increases and narrows the gap between the power of the professional and the dependence of the patient.

Medicine is unable to control and restrain the right of 'alternative' providers, such as complementary medicine.

In presenting the results of this research, the chapter will primarily discuss evidence on the first three of the threats quoted from Hafferty.

It has been stated that one key target of this chapter will be to contextualise the data in the economic and political changes occurring in the U.K. healthcare scene. McKinlay (1988) argues that much healthcare research overlooks the political and economic setting which is essential to understand the 'business of medicine today'. According to Larkin (1988), up to date, medical dominance in the U.K. can be seen as state supported, but also state limited. It is interesting to question if the introduction of an internal market in healthcare will erode the influence of the state?

Finally, the role of a clinical manager actively engaged in guiding the service and colleagues challenges the collegiality of the profession. It may also redraw the boundaries of individual professional autonomy. Rueschemeyer (1986) discusses why professional managers are rarely featured in the literature of the sociology of professions. Some authors have debated the relative importance of the issue of professional autonomy at both the individual and the collective levels (Wolinsky 1988; Harrison and Schultz, 1989) whilst others (Goode, 1960; Hetherington, 1982) have debated the conflicts between professionalism, professional autonomy and management. As much of the literature is premised on the conflicts between professional and bureaucratic approaches, it adopts the view that any professional moving into management, moves out of the profession. This perspective is clearly open to dispute. However, the research evidence will illustrate that the language of confrontation, using terms such as 'betrayal' and 'desertion' are still employed to exert social pressure on clinical managers.

The key changes affecting doctors

In order to create an internal market in healthcare, through the NHS and Community Care Act 1990, purchasers and providers have to be separated. Then, at the core of a process of contracting for healthcare delivery is the ability to specify a level of service from a group of clinicians and other paramedics, to a specified cost and quality. This is one of the main impetus for involving clinicians actively in management decisions. It is virtually impossible to imagine how managers, in isolation, could carry out the tasks required to specify the type, form, quality standards and volumes of a specific medical service without the active involvement of the clinical specialists.

The NHS and Community Care Act also specifies the inclusion of clinicians in the management process in a more particular way. A place is reserved for a medical specialist on the boards of both Trusts and FHSAs. This gives clinicians access to the most senior and strategic decision making forums.

In addition to the effects of the NHS and Community Care Act, there is a vast amount of service change underway at the unit level. Some of these changes are themselves part of substantial shifts in the way service is provided eg the policy to move the majority of mentally ill patients from institutional settings into the community. The range of changes and the processes of implementation are documented and analysed elsewhere (Pettigrew et al., 1992; Harrison, 1988) and will not be dealt with here. The background to this discussion therefore is one of major and transformational change in the healthcare sector.

The impact of the changes on individuals

The first and most notable impact of the recent changes on individual clinicians is that many more of them have accepted medical management roles, either as clinical directors or as medical directors. Historically, doctors have been reluctant to move into management roles. (Stewart, undated; FitzGerald and Sturt, 1992). The Griffiths report (1983) stated that a crucial target for the health service was to encourage more doctors into general management. On the whole, after the initial publicity, there was no sustained flow. One reason for this was the discrepancies of pay, but it can be argued that another equally important reason was that general management was a full-time commitment. Few doctors were willing to make this irrevocable move. Finally, there were subtle social and status reasons. Stewart's (undated) work demonstrates the mistrust doctors had of managers and the oft-held belief that managers had completely alien values.

As a result of Griffiths, the advent of general management did introduce considerable changes in the management processes, which may have provided an added impetus to doctors' current acceptance of management roles. Power shifted more towards managers, either directly as a result of budgetary control and resource constraints inducing change; or indirectly through such changes as the introduction of new information technology.

Currently, the motivation of clinicians to move into management is based in a complex judgement of a number of interacting factors. Nevertheless, the outcome is that large numbers of doctors are becoming clinical managers either as clinical directors heading a service or as medical directors managing a trust. A recent survey (Harwood and Boufford, 1993) shows that in 75 per cent of the directorates studied, the clinical director's post was held by a doctor. The factors influencing individual's decisions to become a clinical manager emanate from the contextual or environmental, organizational and individual levels. It is the combination of these factors which appears to have caused the clinicians to alter their past judgements and accept a management role.

Key to these altered judgements are the assessments that members of the cohort are making about the changing face of healthcare in the U.K. Consultants in the cohort expressed a range of views about the impact of the NHS and Community Care Act 1990. Despite differing political leanings, the majority of people saw the changes as fundamental and likely to have long term impact on healthcare. (This finding holds though initial interviews took place both before and after the last General Election.) One clinician described his expectations of the impact of the Act in this way:

> We'll be able to sharpen up our priorities and we shall be able to present much more clearly to health authorities, and this is what I think we should be doing, a choice about how they spend their money on behalf of the public. And they can choose between so many hips, at such a price compared with developments in the community or dealing with the emergency workload.

All the cohort wanted to influence the direction or form of change and could foresee opportunities to do this in their new role. These findings differ from those emerging from other current research (Dopson, 1995; Dawson at al., 1995) and demonstrate that the cohort under study are particularly positive in their view of their management role. This can be explained by the careful selection and screening of individuals entering this management training programme. All participants had studied management (if only superficially) and the majority of them have agreed to accept a management role willingly. When compared with an alternative cohort also undertaking management training (Dopson, 1995), it can be seen that some clinicians are accepting management roles more reluctantly, because they feel that someone must take on the tasks or that a clinician is a better choice than a manager.

At the organizational level, the challenge of management is reinforced by the nature of the part-time job on offer. Most of the clinicians in the cohort wish to maintain their clinical role and continue to practise as a doctor. A minority of doctors in the cohort were contemplating moving into management in the long term, though none of them wished to give up their clinical practice immediately.

One of the clearest and most uniform findings to emerge from the study is personal motivation at the individual level. The stimulation and interest of a new challenge is a powerful motivator to doctors. Time after time, consultants used virtually identical words to explain why they had decided to take on a management role.

> It's a challenging role I have. I've looked at it this way, that there are not many people who get the opportunity to start a new career at the age of fifty, which I have and I find this to be very stimulating.

The career structures in the medical profession mean that there are new hurdles which have to be overcome every two/three years as one progresses towards a consultant position. Once this is achieved, the individual faces twenty to thirty years in the same role, with few new challenges.

The data referred to so far demonstrate that the current changes are causing a reassessment by the clinicians in the cohort. To understand the basis of these evaluations, one has to take account of the combination of factors acting together. Some of these factors, such as the challenge of a new role are not new, but are now viewed differently against other factors. Similarly, the assessments are better understood when viewed against the historical backcloth. Many of the clinicians in the cohort referred to their past experiences and concluded that the medical profession should have more influence on management decision making.

The second major impact on individuals is the opportunity to hold a position with real influence and decision making power in the broader organisational arena. This statement is not intended to imply that clinical decisions do not involve the exercise of power, but to recognise that clinical managers are operating in the organizational arena.

The individual clinicians in the cohort all faced the need to manage substantial and often multiple changes in the provision of services. It was not unusual for a clinical manager to describe his/her work demands in terms of two or three major changes. Typically, these might include the relocation or expansion of a service to a new site; the adoption of different technology to deliver services and the reskilling of staff or the reconfiguration of skills to provide more effective use of resources. Clinical managers therefore defined the demands of their roles in terms of high levels of strategic and service change and the need for change management. To quote one clinical director:

> As a theatre manager, I am developing an internal contract with surgical users, but I am frustrated by the lack of reliable information. Also, I am managing a major change caused by the rebuilding programme in theatres.

However, the reality of these demands are not always accurately reflected in the job descriptions held by Clinical Directors.

From the analysis of their work, one can conclude that the clinical management role involves considerable amounts of change management and strategic management. There is thus the opportunity to exercise influence and participate in decision making. Many professionals are now budget holders and are responsible for major spending decisions. Clinical Directors also have a key role to play in agreeing contracts and in service development. The evidence suggests that, with the appropriate training, clinical managers can rapidly develop their approach to strategic planning in a competitive context. One Clinical Director described the consultative processes which had been adopted within his/her directorate to draw up a strategic plan. These processes included two away-days for the executive team. Their work had culminated in the definition of the key objective for the speciality 'to be one of the top ten units (in their speciality) in the UK in the next five years.' More significantly, the operational criteria for defining a 'top' unit had been specified by reference to bench marks, drawn against data from other similar units in the U.K. Meetings were being held with Dutch doctors developing a similar management approach.

In the second study, the evidence (Ferlie, FitzGerald & Ashburner 1992; Ferlie, Ashburner & FitzGerald, 1993) suggests that Medical Directors (and their colleagues representing teaching hospitals) in Trusts and Public Health Directors on Health Authorities are exercising considerable influence on boards. In the majority of boards studied, medical directors and directors of public health were active participants on the boards. Medical Directors occupied positions of considerable influence on a number of the boards studied, where their views on medical/medical related matters were deferred to. Moreover, in a number of examples medical directors were allowed to be more challenging and express dissident views. It can be argued that for any board to work effectively, a balance has to be struck between homogeneity and the danger of 'group-think' and diverse views and the danger of non-agreement. In the private sector, Cadbury (1992) has argued that:

an essential quality which NEDs should bring to the board's deliberations is that of independence of judgement.

Whilst some boards studied exhibited great homogeneity and low levels of dissent, in others there appeared to be 'licensed dissenters' operating. For this form of dissent to be accepted and listened to, dissenters had to have high self confidence, adopt a subtle approach to raising issues and have a secure base within the system. Medical Directors and Directors of Public Health were regularly found in this challenging role.

On the positive side therefore, it is clear that these clinical management roles offer members of the medical profession the opportunity to take and participate in major decisions, affecting the delivery of healthcare. Moreover, both the clinical directors and especially the medical directors have new spheres of influence as members of the Trust board or Trust executive. In this way, they have access to the highest level management discussions and are involved at the start in the process of planning changes. With the advent of general management, power could be seen to have shifted towards management and these new senior roles redress the balance in favour of the medical profession. They offer an opportunity to develop genuinely collaborative decision making processes and structures, so long as clinicians can be found with the willingness and managerial capacity to engage in healthcare management.

On the other hand, it is apparent that there are negative aspects to the current situation. Further thought may be needed to define the part-time clinical manager's role in the most effective way possible. This is likely to mean a continuing period of role refinement and renegotiation. Many clinical managers are currently coping with an overload of work. Therefore the configuration and quality of support staff is a vital dimension of these developments. A recent survey (Harwood & Boufford, 1993) stresses the critical importance of the clinical management team for the effective operation of clinical management. There is evidence of major problems in the appropriate selection and training of clinical managers. Whilst the results of this project demonstrate that it is possible to address these issues constructively, the data also suggest that priority has to be given to clinical management training; resources dedicated to it and an infrastructure put in place that allows training to be organised economically and effectively.

The impact of the quasi-market on professional boundaries

One of the questions raised by the advent of the quasi-market is how clinical managers would relate to general managers and how they would relate to their own medical colleagues. Clinical managers are an extreme example of specialists moving into a corporate or generalist role. As a profession, medicine is academically orientated. Doctors' perceptions of management and what management entails are coloured by their contact with managers in healthcare and by the frequently held view that managers are not well qualified and management is easy to learn.

The clinicians in this cohort are unusual in that they all had prior management training, even if this was only a few days' course. Similarly they all had experience of management. Nevertheless, their perceptions of 'management' were still relatively unsophisticated. At the start of the study, the majority of the cohort described management in terms of a set of skills which frequently focussed on 'people' skills, such as appraising, selecting, and performance management. In practice, such perceptions mean that even with goodwill and a motivation to learn more about management, there is still a gulf of experience and knowledge to bridge. (It should be noted that this is a two-way problem with some managers believing in the stereotypes of doctors.)

In this cohort, clinicians went to programmes of management training based in high quality business schools and undertook intensive courses for middle or senior managers alongside participants from all sectors of business.

It is notable that following the period of study, there is a shift in the clinicians' perceptions of management and more particularly, the areas of management learning which might prove most useful to them in the future. For some, there is the revelation of discovering a functional area of management, which proves to be relevant to their own management problems. For others, it is the recognition that management issues in healthcare are repeated, albeit in a different form, in other organisations. A quote will exemplify:

> I think it was the emphasis on quality as the concern of everyone i.e. that we are all a customer of each other, interdepartmentally. That struck me most. And the positive emphasis on welcoming complaints and dealing with them. All of these things are quite radical and different concerns from those we are used to in the NHS.

After training, clinical managers frequently mentioned the areas of management which are outward looking and deal with the interfaces between the whole organization and it's competitors, customers and suppliers as particularly relevant to their roles. These topics would normally be described in terms of strategic management, marketing and business policy. Clinicians stressed the conceptual development of thinking about the NHS as a business, albeit a 'not-for-profit' business. The overwhelming reaction of the cohort members to their training was positive. Unanimously, consultants saw the programmes as beneficial, and were particularly supportive of the opportunity to mix and learn with managers form other sectors. A majority of the cohort stated that they had gained confidence as a consequence of their training. These positive findings are reinforced by the results from a broader national sample (Cowling and Newman, 1994).

Once back in their role as a clinical manager, the data provide evidence of a consistent process of applying learning within the management role. To give some diverse examples, cohort members are involved in the restructuring of medical staffing; in drawing up a strategic plan for a newly created Family Planning and Women's Health Service and in marketing to GPFHs. Clinical managers state that through increased confidence and knowledge, they are better able to understand and to question other managers. Some illustrations of the comments made:

> I have more confidence in asking the right questions; identifying expertise and ways of solving problems, as a result of attendance on the programme. I am more 'system-wise', I have a wider appreciation of organisation.

> I walked around with a perpetual feeling of guilt, if I was doing management work, I felt I should be doing medicine and vice versa. Now I see the importance of the management side, I've got that sorted out and I delegate!

As demonstrated in the previous section, the role played by Medical Directors within the Trust board is both influential and critical. A medical director in the cohort described the role as 'a bridging role' between management and the medics. Another stated:

> The ability of the Chair, the CEO and the Medical Director on a board to communicate very closely is essential.

All the evidence from both studies reinforces the validity of this statement. In boards which worked effectively as teams, there was open and constructive debate and communication between the executives and the non-executives. Where boards were seen to be developing and progressing the service strategy for the Trust, active and credible Medical Directors were one component of this success. To play this part adequately, one Medical Director suggested:

> My view is if you are going to put someone in a senior corporate role, like medical director, they need to go away to mixed group courses. [i.e. to courses where participants are from mixed backgrounds and are not a uni-professional group.]

These data illustrate an influential role being played by this cohort of clinicians once they have gained greater knowledge of management and more confidence in their management abilities.

The evidence also suggests that Clinical Managers are grasping some thorny problems, in relation to medical colleagues and dealing with issues which have been allowed to fester up to now. There are two particular aspects of their management experience which will be explored in more detail here. Firstly, clinicians describe embarking on the resolution of problems, sometimes of long standing, in relation to their clinical colleagues. These are issues relating to differential levels of performance among colleagues, as well as inequitable distribution of workload. Up till the present, clinical freedom has meant that few General Managers dared to deal with these issues. These problems of performance may be broached via the processes of medical audit. The problems in relation to workload and the distribution of work may be currently highlighted by the need to alter junior doctors' hours of work, but this also provides a lever to address the issues. Significantly, it appears that there are some indicators here that issues of professional performance and professional standards are being addressed and handled by clinical managers.

A second feature of the clinical management role focussed on by clinicians was the nature of their relationships with other doctors. They stated that where they are experiencing difficulties in their management roles, these are frequently linked to problems of relationships with colleagues, either management or medical.

Members of the cohort described their current priorities as centering on interpersonal relations;

> I am using the course learning in the way I am dealing with difficult people. ....This especially helps in dealings with junior doctors/ consultants. I have learnt how to say 'No'.

All the clinical managers see themselves playing a critical boundary role between management and the medical professionals. They describe part of their role as 'translating' ideas from one forum to the other. Several members of the cohort commented on the importance of not exhibiting too much 'missionary' zeal on management topics, as this would have a dysfunctional effect on some colleagues.

Whilst many clinical managers experience support from colleagues and managers, there are some who see themselves as separated and on occasion, isolated from clinical colleagues. The extent of this isolation varies considerably from one location to another. In some instances, it is merely a question of occasionally employing management terms which are not understood by medical colleagues.

> I do feel at quite a distance, mentally, from most of my colleagues. I have to frame what I say to colleagues in an acceptable form; I cannot use the language that I have in common with managers, of cost and resources. Over the course of the last year, I have changed quite a lot.....

In other examples, clinical managers are subjected to a degree of downright hostility from some colleagues which causes stress.

In the medium term the willingness of consultants to take on clinical management roles may be influenced by these events and pressures. To quote one Medical Director:

> If I decide to leave this role, it will be because of the isolation and the sense of distance from colleagues.

(and this was a setting where both professional colleagues and managers were on the whole supportive).

If high quality, experienced clinical managers are to be recruited and retained, then these are issues of concern.

Conclusions

Any conclusions from this study must be tentative because of the size of the cohort. Furthermore, the clinicians involved in the study are a skewed group of clinicians who are interested in management and wish to influence management decisions. It is notable that such a group exists and can be replicated in every other Region.

In considering the impact of the current changes on individual clinicians, one key external factor is the manner in which the NHS and Community Care Act has changed the way healthcare is now being delivered. Clinicians have reassessed an interrelated set of factors and the result has been a significant shift in moving clinicians into management.

The response of clinicians to the changed circumstances is to adapt. This response is at once opportunistic and proactive. Clinicians in the group are motivated by a desire to influence the form of care provided and in some cases, to improve on the way decisions have been taken in the past. They are also motivated by career ambition, against the background of a changed organizational setting, where many believe that commercial skills will become more rather than less important. The speed and capability of adaptation is characteristic of the profession.

In this changed context, clinicians in the cohort are assuming new and powerful managerial roles as clinical directors and as medical directors. These roles provide the chance to influence decisions about the service or business plan of each directorate and overall to participate in decisions about the allocation of resources. The role of Medical Director gives guaranteed access to senior management discussions. These changes, it may be argued, potentially considerably strengthen the sphere of influence of the medical profession vis a vis management. They offer access to decision making fora which were not guaranteed prior to the Act. In this respect, the evidence in the U.K. seems to support the thesis put forward by Freidson (1987) in the USA, that the medical profession collectively has not lost it's position of dominance, but has adapted to suit changing circumstances.

It is apparent that within the current context the relationships between clinical managers and general managers have the potential to alter and improve. However the realisation of this potential is dependent on equipping both parties with the understanding and the skill to work with each other. The issue of appropriate training is a particularly high priority for clinical managers since fewer of them have prior management training or experience. The potential for conflict, if the relationships are not handled effectively, is evident in the small number of high profile crisis cases reported in the press, e.g. the vote of 'no confidence' in the Chair by a group of clinicians at Brighton Health Trust.

The evidence suggests that relationships with other doctors produce both threats and benefits. The threats lie in the difficult relationships and isolation which a number of clinical managers have to face. This may inhibit the development of collaborative and productive 'hybrid' roles. The data illustrate that where clinical managers are addressing longstanding issues of quality audit and performance standards, there is a danger that rifts between the managers and the managed will increase, as Hafferty (1988) predicted. Much will depend on the views of the majority of the profession and whether they support the need for such developments. It may be judged that a more unpalatable alternative would be the imposition of centrally driven standards, or greater managerial intervention.

Some clinical managers may be further distanced from their colleagues as their understanding and use of management concepts increases. At least initially, this is likely to generate some dissent within the ranks of the profession.

If one shifts the level of analysis, it can be seen that at the inter organizational level, contracting for services and the quasi-market may have other consequences for professionals. Whilst at the unit level, it can be demonstrated that individual clinicians have gained positions of influence; it can also be argued that competition between Trusts is growing and that this constitutes competition within the medical profession itself. As the specification of contracts increases in precision and the information systems supporting contracting improve, so one is able to distinguish the distinctive competencies of a particular service. Differences of performance in terms of volume and quality of outcomes are exposed. This may help the purchasers to discriminate between services, but it is also a fundamental challenge to the collegiality of the profession which is premised on the equality of professionals. It is this aspect of the changes which many in the profession dislike. Thus, there are early indicators that the 'threat' expounded by Hafferty (1988) of an internal market introducing competition between professionals may have some foundation.

Finally, the jury is still out on whether the introduction of the quasi-market will reduce the central control of the State. The policy of introducing market-like mechanisms could be explained as an attempt to curb professional powers by introducing mediating devices and delegating rationing decisions. However, many professionals felt that one desirable feature of the Trusts was their relative freedom from Regional and central bureaucratic control. This autonomy and freedom has proved rather ephemeral and with the latest changes to newly configured Regional Offices, the regulatory framework is still clearly in transition.

References

Ashburner, L., Ferlie, E. and Fitzgerald, L. (1993), *'Leadership by Boards in Healthcare'* Research for Action Paper 12, Bristol, NHSTD.

Bell, D. (1973), *The Coming of Post-Industrial Society*, New York, Basic Books.

Cadbury Report (1992), *'Report on the Committee on the Financial Aspects of Corporate Governance'*, London, Gee Publishing.

Cowling, A. and Newman, K. (1994), 'Turning doctors into managers: an evaluation of a major NHS initiative to improve the managerial capabilities of medical consultants', *Human Resource Management Journal*, Vol.4, No.4, Summer, 1-14.

Davies, C. (1983), 'Professionals in Bureaucracies: The Conflict Thesis Revisited', in Dingwall, R. and Lewis, P. *The Sociology of the Professions*, London, Macmillan.

Dawson, S. et al. (1995), 'In or out of management? Dilemmas and developments in Public Health Medicine in England', in Leopold, J., Glover, I. and Hughes, M. (eds), *Beyond Reason?*, Avebury, Aldershot.

Dopson, S. (1995), 'Doctors in management: A challenge to established debates', in Leopold, J., Glover, I. and Hughes, M. (eds), *Beyond Reason?*, Avebury, Aldershot.

Ferlie, E., FitzGerald, L. and Ashburner, L. (1992), *'The Challenge of Purchasing'* Research for Action Paper 7, Bristol, NHSTD.

Ferlie, E., Ashburner, L. and FitzGerald, L. (1993), *'Board Teams: Roles and Relationships'* Research for Action Paper 10, Bristol, NHSTD.

FitzGerald, L. (1993), *Management Development for Consultants: Formative Evaluation of the Doctors in Business Schools Programme. Final Report* Unpublished Report. Trent RHA/Department of Health.

FitzGerald, L. and Sturt, J. (1992), 'Clinicians into Management: on the Change Agenda or Not?' *Health Services Management Research* 5/2: 137-146.

Freidson, E. (1984), The Changing Nature of Professional Control, *Annual Review of Sociology* 10:1-20.

Freidson, E. (1986), *Professional Powers: a Study of the Institutionalisation of Formal Knowledge,* University of Chicago Press.

Freidson, E. (1987), 'The Future of the Professions', *Journal of Dental Education* 53: 140-144

Goode, W.J. (1960), Community within a community: the professions, *American Sociological Review*, Vol. 22, No. 194.

Griffiths Report (1983), *Report of the NHS Management Inquiry*, (D83) 38, London, HMSO.

Hafferty, Frederic (1988), Theories at the Crossroads: A Discussion of Evolving Views on Medicine as a Profession, *The Millbank Quarterly* 66/2 :202-225.

Harrison, Stephen (1988), *Managing the National Health Service, Shifting the Frontier?* London, Chapman and Hall.

Harrison, S. and Schultz, R. I. (1989), Clinical Autonomy in the U.K. and the U.S.A.: contrasts and convergence, in Freddi, G. & Bjorkman, J.W. (eds), *Controlling Medical Professionals*, London, Sage.

Harwood, A. and Boufford, I. J. (1993), *Managing Clinical Services: A consensus statement of principles for effective clinical management*, BAMM; BMA; IHSM; RCN.

Hetherington, R. H. (1982), Quality Assurance and Organisational Effectiveness in Hospitals, *Health Services Management Research*, Vol. 17, No. 2.

Larkin, G. V. (1988), Medical Dominance in Britain: Image and Reality, *The Millbank Quarterly* 66/2 : 117-132.

McKinlay, B. (1988), Introduction: The Changing Character of the Medical Profession, *The Millbank Quarterly* 66/2 : 1-9.

N.H.S. and Community Care Act (1991), London: HMSO.

Pettigrew, A., Ferlie, E. and McKee, L. (1992), *Shaping Strategic Change: the case of the NHS*, London, Sage.

Prahalad, C.K. and Hamel, G. (1990), The Core Competency of the Corporation, *Harvard Business Review*, May-June, 79-91.

Reuschemeyer, D. (1986) ,*Power and the Division of Labour*, *Polity Press*.

Senge, P. (1991), *The Fifth Discipline* New York, Random Books.

Stewart, Rosemary (undated), *Involving Doctors in General Management*.

Templeton Series, Paper 5, Bristol, NHSTA.

Wolinsky, F. D. (1988), The Professional dominance perspective re-visited, *The Millbank Quarterly*, 66:2, 33-47.

Zuboff, S. (1988), *In the Age of the Smart Machine*, London, Heinemann.

PART IV

RATIONALIZATION

11 The role of clinicians in the management of the NHS

Lynn Ashburner

Introduction

The profession of medicine and its conceptual framework have developed and changed as a consequence of many challenges over a long history. These challenges have come from a variety of sources, for example, from government, from within the profession, from allied professional groups and, within an organizational setting, from management. The recent challenge from the growth of managerialism within the NHS needs to be analyzed to understand the extent to which the changes now occurring fall within this process of continuing adaptation or whether they represent a more significant shift in the balance of power between the profession and management. It is far too simplistic to view managers and medical professionals as two distinct, opposed groups. This chapter examines the bases of medicine's professional power by analysing research findings to show how old inter and intra professional boundaries are changing and how new relationships are developing which have led to changes in the professions power base. This raises the important question of whether such new bases of power can be accounted for within the traditional concept of a 'profession' or whether the concept itself needs to be developed.

The development of all professions can be traced through the process of establishing and defending their boundaries; through attempts at closure and the monopolising of specific applications of knowledge. In one sense what the profession faces in the 1990s is a continuation of this process but there are features of the present challenge which differ from those in the past. Firstly there is the context of the NHS and public sector restructuring process which has been the major policy objective of the Conservative government since the early 1980s and secondly, there is the challenge of the growth of new and other expert groups, such

207

as management. In organizational settings, such as the NHS, where professional power has traditionally been dominant, the possibility that managerialism might not only successfully reduce important aspects of medical power but also whether it is feasible that it might replace medicine as the dominant group, needs to be carefully analyzed. The 'control' of the medical profession is a more complex issue than that for other professions given the centrality of the concept of 'medical autonomy'. Current theoretical thinking on the issue of medical autonomy will be examined in relation to the research data. Trends in the UK can be compared with those in the US where some writers have suggested that a process of deprofessionalisation (Haug, 1973) or proletarianisation (McKinlay and Arches, 1985) is occurring. In this context, the process of change currently being experience within the NHS makes the question of what are the limits to managerialism, critical.

The data for this chapter are drawn from a three year research project which was designed to examine the effects of the 1990 health service reforms at the level of the authority, board and senior management. The methodology was designed to combine qualitative and survey methods. A postal questionnaire was sent to all health authority and trust members in 1990-91, which showed the extent of the professional presence on these bodies. The qualitative component consisted of eleven intensive and longitudinal case studies which comprised: two regional health authorities (RHAs), three district health authorities (DHAs), two family health service authorities (FHSAs) and four acute trusts, (two first, one second and one third wave), to form nested hierarchies. Board members and other key stakeholders including senior clinicians were interviewed. The analysis of the data focuses on both the relationship between doctors and managers and that between different parts of the profession, which may respond in different ways.

The medical profession and the growth of managerialism

Historically the focus of power within the health service has lain with doctors. At the formation of the NHS in 1948 as Harrison and Schultz (1989) point out, the government guaranteed the medical profession autonomy to ensure their participation in the newly formed health service. The day to day running of the service was carried out by administrators and, as Elston (1991) shows in her analysis of the development of medical power, it was not until the 1970s that there was any effective challenge to the medical profession's position. This was despite several processes of restructuring. Such attempts at increasing managerial control in the NHS were judged by Klein (1984) to have fallen victim to medical power. The impetus for reform was a concern over rising costs and lack of accountability in the use of resources.

The new 1979 Conservative government had a strong commitment to reducing public expenditure. There was an added pressure in most western economies of a reducing GDP and the modest contribution of medicine to the health status of populations (McKinlay, 1988). The government's chosen means of controlling expenditure were to reduce expansion, cut costs and improve managerial performance. In the name of efficiency, the power of both the growing bureaucracies and the professional groups within them, were explicitly or implicitly being challenged.

The introduction of line management after the Griffiths enquiry (1983), was an attempt to introduce private sector models, structures and personnel to the NHS. Griffiths also recommended that doctors should be brought into management but this never became a key government objective. This structural approach to reform was seen by writers such as Cox (1991) as an inappropriate solution, since the NHS resembled less a bureaucracy than a loosely structured order with complex sets of relationships between administrators and professional groups, as described by Burns (1981). Previous studies of reform in the NHS have found a very high degree of cultural resilience and minimal actual change (Elcock, 1978) and this is what the 'new' managers also found. However successful or not the Griffiths initiative was deemed to be, it had the laid the foundation for the subsequent reforms.

Whether the challenge came from government or other professional groups, the British medical profession had proved adept at resisting change and major inroads with regard to its level of autonomy. Halpern (1992) shows how by the use of political and institutional processes, the medical profession has remained dominant over allied professions, throughout all its interprofessional struggles. In this it has been reliant upon the government to continue to legitimise its monopoly of certain medical procedures. The present challenge, from government itself, may be more difficult to withstand.

The latest health service reforms are the consequence of a review announced in early 1988. Unlike any preceding review, this one was carried out without the formal inclusion of the Royal Colleges and the BMA (Elston, 1991). The subsequent white paper *Working for Patients* (DoH, 1989), introduced a range of policies which would affect all parts of the service. The central premise was that the roles of purchaser and provider should be separated and that the mechanisms of health care provision should be governed by an internal or quasi-market, rather than by local and central planning. This included the option for many sub-organisational units of going for trust status to secure a degree of autonomy. Although this raised the greatest controversy politically, concern within the medical profession was equally focused on the introduction of GP fundholders. Under this scheme GPs would be allowed to hold the budgets for a range of patient services and purchase these direct from providers, giving the government the potential to introduce cash limits on GP's expenditure.

The least publicised aspect of the reforms was the changes to the composition of health authorities and the newly created trusts, which were based upon the private sector board of directors model. Old style authorities which comprised twenty plus professional, lay and local authority members were replaced by bodies of just eleven, five of whom, for the first time, were to be senior managers (Ashburner and Cairncross, 1993). The new style authorities specifically exclude professionals with a representational role. There is a statutory place for just one medical practitioner on trust boards as an executive member, and for one GP on FHSAs, until they are merged with DHAs, but no places on RHAs or DHAs. These latter are forming the basis of the new purchasing organizations.

Structurally it would appear that medical involvement, and that of other health professionals, has been greatly reduced. As authorities and boards increasingly are being seen as more effective strategic decision making bodies (Ashburner, Ferlie and FitzGerald, 1993), then the loss of representation of medical and other health service professionals, could be significant. In reality the relative position of professionals in relation to management is more complex, with the development of clinical management teams, clinical directorates and the medical director post within provider units and the growing emphasis on public health expertise in the purchasing units. In the primary sector the introduction of GP fundholders has given a growing groups of doctors a completely new set of powers. By holding their own budgets, GPs can decide which provider units to contract with. A key outcome of this has been that the relationship between GPs and hospital doctors has been fundamentally altered.

This continuing emphasis on the growth of managerialism has changed the existing relationships and power bases within the NHS, with doctors being those potentially most affected. As Ashburner, Ferlie and FitzGerald (1995) show, the large number and the ideological rather than the structural nature of the reforms, plus the persistence of government focus, has created a situation which differs from the past both in the processes which are ongoing and the direction in which they are moving.

The theoretical context

If the profession of medicine is undergoing significant change, it is necessary to understand the importance of the concepts of medical autonomy and medical dominance which are central to their development as a profession and whether, with the rise of managerialism, these central tenets are under serious threat. There have been several theoretical approaches to the study of the professions and these do not always agree on what should be included in an analysis of a profession. The functionalist tradition with its emphasis on the defining features of a profession cannot aid an analysis of differentials in the distribution of power, control and rewards within a profession. As Atkinson and Delamont (1990) show, to limit an analysis in this way merely uncritically reproduces the professionals own claims and over emphasises the degree of homogeneity within the profession. There needs to be several dimensions to an analysis with a distinction needing to be made between the individual power of a professional and their collective power. Equally, as Murray, Dingwall and Eekelaar (1983) show a distinction needs to be made between the 'outward' and 'inward' faces of a profession. The 'outward' view focuses on professions as neutral, knowledge based and working for the 'general good', but for the analysis to turn inward, requires a very different set of concepts.

An alternative starting point, from the interactionist tradition, places the professions as falling within a general classification of occupations, with any differences between groups being of degree rather than kind. By looking at the internal characteristics of occupations, such theorists would dispute the level of homogeneity that is assumed by functionalists and draw attention to the exchange relationships which exist both within a profession and between related professions, which result in differential distributions of power, rewards and control. The second of these approaches offers more scope for increasing understanding but neither places the professions in their social, political, economic and historical contexts.

In the study of the medical profession, many writers have attempted to remedy this with analyses rooted in a social context (McKinlay, 1988; Abbott, 1988; Hafferty, 1988); in a political, economic, gender and race context (Davies, 1983; Navarro, 1988; Atkinson and Delamont, 1990); in a historical context (Larkin, 1988; Navarro, 1988); how it impacts on organisational forms (Scott, 1985) and how it is linked into the class and labour market systems (Hall, 1988). Several of these writers have developed ideas which are useful in the present context. Hafferty, for example, suggests that it is not possible to understand the nature of modern professions without relating them to the wider social and economic trends and this is clearly the starting point for the present analysis. Abbott stresses the need to place the study of the professions in their social context and he has developed a dynamic model which sees the professions as part of a system of occupations each with their own jurisdiction, with different levels of control and with boundaries which are in perpetual dispute. For the purposes of the present study a similar analysis could be applied to the relationships within a profession. Scott develops this further by considering the relationship between the two levels of analysis. His analysis considers how environmental changes affect health care organisations and the consequent changes in the relationship between managers and professionals, which has a clear relevance for the present day NHS. What is important is that any analysis focuses attention on the inner and outer contexts of professional systems.

Within this analytical framework, it is necessary to examine the bases of the medical profession's power. This is typically seen as resting upon its formal control of expertise, its monopoly of practice, its control over entry to the profession, its inherent characteristics and societal approbation. These variously contribute to our understanding of the two predominant concepts which are used to assess changes to the status of the medical profession, professional autonomy and professional dominance. The latter refers primarily to the dominance of the medical profession over the work of other related health professionals (Freidson, 1970). Although this is an important dimension in the total calculation of the relative status of a profession it has less relevance for the present study which focuses on the relationship between management and doctors and within the medical profession. It is the concept of professional or medical autonomy which needs to be explored in order that the dimensions of professional power and changes to these can be recognised and their relative importance assessed. The concept of professional autonomy has several dimensions to it, with an important one being the between the individual and the collective. Then there are different aspects of autonomy with economic, political and clinical being the main ones. It is the last of these, also called clinical freedom, which has formed the basis of debate with regard to the increase in managerial power. At the formation of the NHS the medical profession gave up a considerable amount of economic autonomy in order to retain clinical autonomy. This is the concept which best expresses the level of control that the profession exerts at both an individual and collective level over their work. Even so the relative importance ascribed to clinical autonomy by different writers varies considerably, from those such as Wolinsky (1988) who sees it as a 'red herring' to Harrison and Schultz (1989) who see it as being at the heart of the professions debate. This is a problematic area. Wolinsky's point is that clinical autonomy in a pure sense cannot and has never existed; there are always some constraints on medical decision making. Another problem is the extent to which clinical freedom can be used in an emotive way by the profession and its defenders to challenge any changes which have been initiated outside the profession, whether these represent a real challenge or just a change in the way that clinical decisions are made. To be useful the term needs to be used more critically. As with many concepts, it cannot be defined precisely but it can be useful as a measure of the extent of changes which might either enhance or reduce it.

The NHS reforms and the growth of managerialism are not the only changes which might affect the autonomy of the medical profession. Other factors include the growth of clinical audit, increased specialisation, the use of technology, and the growth in allied professions and their continuing aspirations. It is the extent of these challenges which have led theorists in the US to suggest that a process of either deprofessionalisation (Haug, 1973) or proletarianisation (McKinlay and Arches, 1985) is occurring. The deprofessionalisation thesis emphasises the changing relationship between doctors and their patients, with the increase in medical knowledge of those outside the profession. She suggests that medicine's cultural authority is declining and its monopoly of knowledge is under threat. Haug has more recently revised this view (1988) by saying that although individual doctors may be under threat, she sees less impact on the autonomy of the profession collectively.

The proletarianisation thesis is more central to the issues raised by this paper. It suggests that the changing working conditions of doctors and their subordination management and capital, in conjunction with attempts to control their income, have created a fundamental change in their relationship to work. McKinlay and Arches argue that this is an ongoing process where a progressive loss of autonomy and skills with increasing specialization and use of technology, parallels the deskilling process of artisans in the industrial revolution. This is related to the growing bureaucratization of the US health care system with the increasing state control of the financing of health care, and the increase in the corporate provision of health care for profit.

Within the US this view has been challenged by Freidson (1986) who argues that such trends have not led to any clearer articulation of the concept, or assessment of the implications for the professional autonomy of the medical profession; and especially at the collective level, medical power has not been significantly affected. It is important to recognise the differences between the position of the medical profession in the US and Britain. In the US the state has never attempted to control the economic autonomy of doctors, but equally it has never been central to protecting their clinical autonomy, as in Britain. Medical audit and peer review are long established in the US system and controls from the corporate level and insurance companies are increasing as costs continue to escalate (McKinlay and Stoeckle, 1988). Relative to their British counterparts, US doctors are accustomed to far greater intrusions into their clinical autonomy. External controls are likely to impact on the economic autonomy of doctors in the US far more than in Britain where the capacity to control earnings has never been absolute. This lack of government control and protection in the US can be seen to have created the current situation where the clinical and economic autonomy of the medical profession appears to be under greater threat. In Britain where doctors earnings have always been controlled and where large corporations and insurance companies do not control the provision of care, such direct pressures on the medical profession are less likely.

The pressures placed on clinicians in Britain by the growth in managerialism can be assessed in terms of whether and how they impact on medical autonomy but this cannot, as yet, be compared to a process of proletarianisation with its inherent assumption of a one-way process. The emphasis in this study is on the changing relationship between management and the medical profession and the lack of homogeneity within the profession which has resulted in a diverse pattern of medical reactions. It must be stressed that it is too simplistic to see 'management' merely as the agent for the government's reforms; this belies the level of diversity in the health care system and the potentially conflicting interests of different groups of managers.

Clinicians in hospital management

The introduction of clinical directorates as a means of medical management pre-dates the 1990 Act, but the reforms hastened their development. The provisions of the Act for the increased autonomy of hospitals, the need to contract for the provision of health care at the community level and the tightening of budgets were recognised as having extensive implications both for the role of management and of clinicians. As FitzGerald (1995) shows, clinicians made the judgement that these reforms were more significant than in the past and required a different level of response. Prior to the late 1980s there had been considerable resistance from doctors to become involved in management. Although resistance is still present, there has been a rapid growth in the development of clinical directorates.

FitzGerald shows that in two sample regions, three quarters of acute units had established clinical directorates and appointed mainly doctors to the posts of clinical director, by mid 1991.

Managers interviewed in the case study hospitals, all recognised the benefits of the involvement of clinicians in management and many showed a strong desire to increase their involvement. It was recognised that without this involvement, attempts to increase efficiency and effectiveness would be adversely affected. For example, the doctor's role in decision making on admissions and discharge had considerable impact upon the level and use of resources. Even where the doctor's direct control is limited, as with emergency admissions, a medical input is essential for the understanding of the resource implications. Lemieux-Charles's (1992) research in Canada found a positive relationship between high levels of physician-hospital integration and a strong financial performance. The mutual benefits were not seen in purely financial terms by the managers interviewed, most of whom placed the issue of quality of care as of equal importance. Packwood, Keen and Buxton (1992) argue that the mutual benefits of the increased participation of clinicians in management occurred because it brought the work and interests of doctors and managers closer together. Since the new contracting process puts an emphasis on service outputs, the clinical directorate is the ideal structure for assessments and for medical audit, with its collective review of service provision this can increase the perceived level of clinical accountability. The organizational structure of hospitals is important since, as Kinston (1983) argues, this forms the main link between policy and behaviour and it delineates the boundaries and authority relations between groups. Packwood et al. (1992) suggest that what will emerge is a new form of organisation characterised by decentralization, managerial devolution and professional incorporation into management. By involving themselves in management doctors should be in a stronger position to defend their sphere of influence.

The roles of clinical director and medical director are relatively new and there is little research evidence on how these roles are developing. the present research can merely suggest how some clinicians view their role. The medical directors in the study recognised the role conflicts inherent in their role. All the doctors interviewed stressed that their ability to perform their managerial tasks rested upon their retaining their credibility with their medical colleagues and that this was dependent upon their primary role remaining that of practising clinician.

The eight medical and clinical directors interviewed in the two trusts all felt that the clinical directorate system had improved the way that clinicians related to management. Some commented that the increase in the amount and quality of information was important for understanding where the money was spent and in making clinical groups more accountable. Management were seldom seen as imposing decisions and the new structure was considered a vast improvement over the system in operation up to the mid 1980s when, as one clinical director explained, doctors did not know why decisions were being made or who was making them. The development of 'business' plans was also judged to be beneficial in relation to the setting of objectives, the identification of problems and the optimum use of resources, rather than any more direct 'business' objective. This maybe indicates that the terminology in use suggests a more entrepreneurial approach than that actually being taken. One clinical director expressed the view that when managers and clinicians were working together well, the quality of decisions was improved. As another said:

It is now more difficult to sidestep management decisions by going along the professional route; now if doctors are going to retain a say in services they need to get involved in management and put their case forward that way.

However, the relationship between managers and clinicians was still viewed as in need of improvement. Some clinical directors expressed the view that at board level there was not always a real appreciation of what many aspects of medical work involved. The observation of board meetings showed that the members of the board, especially the non-executives, were dependent upon the medical director for information on the medical implications of the issues under discussion. The medical director's ability to take on this corporate role would be likely to vary considerably between individuals. This is a critical communication link which few boards in the study had addressed directly. One clinical director felt that this had led on his trust to some management decisions being seen by clinicians as unrealistic. Another was concerned that some management decisions were not referred to all clinical levels before a decision was reached.

The issues identified as critical were the perceived inequalities between directorates in how their income was calculated in relation to actual work done, how work was to be shared and the question of priority setting. In the latter case one doctor felt that it was still a case of 'who shouted loudest'. Budget cutting at purchaser level fed down to reduced budgets at directorate level and rivalry for funds, between directorates became a fact of life. This led one medical director to state that the skills he needed most were those of leadership and maintaining morale. The dissatisfactions that were voiced by doctors related not just to relationships with managers and between directorates but also with purchasers. The problems that existed with the purchasing authorities might involve agreeing the terms, conditions and most contentiously, the overall size of the contracts, and these frequently served to highlight the constraints within which both management and clinicians were working and very often served to unite doctors with management.

Those doctors interviewed were clearly the 'converts' as they had taken on management roles; and they all referred to the strong sub-group of doctors who refused to become involved in management in any way. Other medical staff were variously described as only being interested in their own directorates or patients, and who thus found it difficult to take a 'corporate' view of what was best for the hospital or community as a whole. Most resistance was believed to come from older doctors and thus the 'problem' was seen as one which experience, education and time would reduce. The major area of conflict between one medical director and his clinical directors, at the time of the study, was in establishing the new arrangements to facilitate the reduction in junior doctors' hours. He added that he would have felt more comfortable in his role had he been elected by his peers rather than having been appointed by the board.

During the first year of the reforms, there was no specific aspect of the 1990 Act which those doctors interviewed could identify as having a direct impact upon their clinical autonomy. It must be remembered, however, that this was the year of 'steady state' instigated by the Department of Health. Several doctors mentioned the Waiting List initiative, which again was Department of Health rather than management sponsored, had been objected to strongly on the basis that admissions were being made on grounds other than clinical need. One clinical director also mentioned that block contracts held with purchasing authorities would have the same outcome, once the pre-set limit to each medical procedure had been reached. Patients of non-fundholding practices would remain on the waiting list whilst those of fundholders would continue to be treated. In subsequent years as the number of GP fundholders increased, discontent with the operation of the internal market increased as this two tier system emerged. If operating theatres and staff capacity were to be fully used and if income to the hospital were to be maintained then managers and doctors faced the uncomfortable prospect of continuing to treat patients of fundholders but not those of non-fundholders. Many doctors and managers disliked the fact that financial rather than clinical need was the criteria for deciding which patients to treat. It must be emphasised that these causes of discontent arose because of the consequences of government policies and not solely as the result of management decisions. In one hospital it was a management decision to continue to treat the patients of non-fundholders on a par with those of fundholders, despite the fact that this 'over-performance' would not be funded.

This type of discontent felt by many doctors may be channelled at management as the conduit of government policy but in essence both groups were equally powerless to change the fundamental inequities that were emerging as a consequence of the reforms. Thus no clear dichotomy of value systems was found in the case study sites, along the management/professional axis. In the survey of the views of health authority and trust members, a significant level of doubt was also expressed about the reforms. For example, on health authorities 46 per cent of managers (i.e. executive rather than non-executive members) disagreed with the statement that 'competition and the internal market would make the NHS more efficient', compared with 72 per cent of chairs (non-executives) who thought it would (Ashburner and Cairncross, 1992). On trusts 60 per cent of chief executives did not believe that trust boards should be modelled on private sector boards, whereas 70 per cent of their chairs did (Ashburner, 1993a). Here is evidence of a clear split between basic value systems but this lies between the executives and non-executives *within* the management hierarchy.

Another clinical director put his views on the increasing influence of management in its wider context:

I do not feel that threatened from a clinical freedom point of view; I do not know whether some of the objections about clinical freedom are a red herring. As regards clinical freedom I have mainly been involved with emergencies and very little elective. I am not clinically free; we deal with it (treatment of patients) in an accepted standard way.

What this suggests is that, given other factors such as agreed protocols for certain treatments, the emergency nature of much of the work and the long history of the waiting list as a rationing device, that clinical freedom in any pure sense has probably never existed, if it is indeed possible. When priorities are judged across all specialities and budgets are limited, these will of necessity constrain clinical decisions. This data suggests that what the increase in the management of service provision has done to date, is to make the rationing decisions more visible, rather than directly increasing the level of control over clinicians. The constraints on clinical practice are the outcome of central policy rather than management decisions.

GP fundholders and non-fundholders

The research included a study of the management role of the FHSA in primary care. General practitioners, as independent contractors in a diffuse system of medical care, cannot be managed directly and so the role of the FHSA has traditionally been one of administration. The 1987 white paper *Promoting Better Health* introduced the new GP contract which was intended to influence the pattern of care provided by GPs to ensure that a wide range of services were more generally available. As Calnan and Gabe (1991) show, it is only in the 1980s that the state has become interested in GPs as a means of controlling expenditure on health care. They add that evaluating the performance of GPs is also in line with the state's policy of attempting to limit the autonomy of certain professional groups.

The 1990 reforms built upon the earlier white paper in extending attempts to manage GPs and introduce fundholding as well as formalising procedures for medical audit and indicative prescribing budgets. FHSAs were given the task of monitoring GPs performance. Thus the role for FHSAs has moved from one of administration to what one general manager called 'management by remote control' (Ashburner, 1993b). What was quickly discovered was that non-fundholding GPs found that their ability to refer patients was now limited mainly to those hospitals where their own DHA had a block contract, whereas GP fundholders could refer wherever they wished.

As highlighted earlier, this two tier system at the level of the GP had an impact upon hospital doctors. In the market system, hospital doctors now found themselves seeking to attract the 'business' of GP fundholders. Clinical directors described the increasing involvement of consultants in the marketing of their services and in negotiations over contracts. This marks a significant shift in power. Calnan and Gabe (1991) describe how GPs have traditionally been viewed within the profession as being of lower status and how this had been shaped by the professional development of hospital medicine. GPs now found hospital clinicians keen to respond to their needs since they now had the power to send patients to other hospitals or to treat them within the primary sector. Another consequence is that non-fundholding GPs without this direct purchasing power have sought to exert more influence upon purchasers to take their needs into account.

This critical change in the balance of power within the medical profession shows how the power and influence of doctors is being affected by forces other than those directly controlled by management. If the increased power of one sector of the medical profession impinges upon another, it might be more problematic for it to be resisted.

A completely new managerial/professional relationship has been created by the increase in fundholding. The greater level of administrative work and the greater size of practices has resulted in the creation of a new role of practice manager. At this stage in the process such managers are the employees of the GPs. Similar issues to those now relating to hospital doctors and their relationship to management will become relevant for GPs. As Pritchard (1987), a practising GP says, the presence of full time professional managers does not mean that GPs can opt out of a management role. He saw the GPs as the directors of the organisation rather than the line managers. Either way the autonomy of the GP fundholder does not appear to be at risk and their actual influence has increased.

Purchasing

The research data on the development of the purchasing function, drawing on data from all three DHAs (Ferlie, FitzGerald and Ashburner, 1992) showed that this had resulted in the increasing prominence of doctors working in public health. One consequence of the reforms, the purchaser provider split, has created the need to contract for services with the result that the work of public health physicians in ascertaining health need for a locality, has become central to the purchasing effort. That this has given public health doctors the potential for greater influence in determining the future shape of health service provision across a wide spectrum, is a factor that has been substantiated by Dawson, Sherval and Mole earlier in this volume. As with GP fundholders this represents an increase in their sphere of influence. Public Health medicine has a chequered history with the changing structures within primary and secondary care having frequently left them marginalised, with constantly changing areas of influence.

In 1988 the Acheson report recommended that a central position needed to be established to act as a focus of effort and that there be a return to the title of Public Health. It recommended that the Director of Public Health should be the chief source of medical advice to the authority and should be part of the key decision making group within the district. The subsequent white paper *Working for Patients* did not, however, provide a statutory place on the new DHAs or purchasing bodies for the Director of Public Health, but merely recommended that authorities should provide themselves with medical and nursing advice. The survey of members carried out in the first year of the new authorities showed that 80 per cent had appointed the Director of Public Health to the board (Cairncross, Ashburner and Pettigrew, 1991), but as on trusts this was into a 'management' role. In all case studies, public health was represented on all the purchasing teams created within the DHAs and the Director of Public Health frequently took a lead in the development of the purchasing role. Their annual report became a key document in the development of strategy.

The role of the public health function in relation to management and in relation to other parts of the medical profession, raises a number of issues. Their role within purchasing is clearly a management role which differs from their traditional role of being a marginal and independent 'thinker', representing the interests of the community. As Dawson et al. argue, this aspect of the reforms may also introduce uncertainty in their future with their loss of 'independence'. On the other hand their role is now central to the process of health needs assessment, rather than being advisory. With a foot in both camps, similar to the position of medical directors on trusts, the possible role conflicts need to be recognised. If however it brings the two perspectives closer together, then this should be beneficial.

The inclusion of the public health role into management will also have an effect on how public health physicians relate to medical professionals in other parts of the service. There are recognised differences of interest and emphasis between the identification of health need on a communal and individual level that relate to how priorities are formed and what comprises the 'greater good'. Initiatives such as the 'Health of the Nation' and the setting of health targets help to determine priorities for provision in purchasing plans. Given their different focus on health need to that of their colleagues who are in direct contact with patients, they may be perceived as being on the management side of any negotiations that take place. Given the dependence of the provider units on contracts from purchasers, this is a second example of a change in the relative balance of power between two groups within the medical profession.

Implications for the balance of power between medical professionals and management

The recent NHS reforms with their continuing emphasis on managerialism can be seen to be a major challenge to the status of the medical profession in the NHS. Given the fundamental way that the reforms are affecting all parts of the NHS, the impact on doctors needs to be understood. The medical profession has enjoyed a high level of professional autonomy and by focusing on changes in their relationships with key external groups such as managers, any changes to their autonomy can begin to be assessed.

It was established earlier that the degree of status and autonomy enjoyed by a profession is the outcome of a combination of factors. What is relevant in one context, such as economic autonomy in the US, is not relevant in others. As Elston (1991) argues, the NHS has shown that salaried status and state intervention are not incompatible with a high level of some aspects of professional autonomy. If it the case that not all aspects are necessarily prerequisites, then it must surely be the case that reductions in the level of one or even a number of defining criteria, need not necessarily impact on the overall assessment of professional status if there is realignment in other areas. Most of the theses about challenges to professional status where the focus is on wider social, political and economic changes have assumed that these must invariably impact in a negative way on the profession, but they have produced little empirical evidence of how this becomes manifest.

The data from this study suggests that the impact of external changes are met not in any simple negative way but with a process of adaption that may in fact change the way that power or autonomy is expressed. The clinical directorate system is a way for clinicians to become involved in management without having to give up clinical practice. There are considerable problems in conceptualising any of the changes which are occurring in terms of either decline or increase in power, given the existence of both. There is a need for a new conceptual framework to emerge.

In this process, an underlying assumption that needs to be challenged is that professionalisation and bureaucratization, as represented by increasing managerialism, are necessarily opposing forces or even alternatives. Hafferty (1988) has shown that bureaucracies can and do make accommodations to professionals and Davies (1983) argues that bureaucracies and professionals can work well together. Scott (1985) suggests that the growth of management influence is partly the result of the needs of the medical profession's increasing complexity and consequent need for co-ordination and management. As organisational environments become more complex and as medical specialities develop, there is a requirement that the range of different interests and the boundaries both internal and external, need greater co-ordination.

The research data from the acute units showed a considerable level of co-operation and acknowledgement of mutual benefit from management and doctors working together. Any increase in the numbers and role of management has, at this stage at least, had a minimal effect directly on the level of clinical autonomy of medical staff. This is making a clear distinction between the effects of the new policies brought in by the reforms, which management have no choice but to implement or which are out of management's control, such as the effects of GP fundholding. The clinical autonomy of medical staff has always been subject to external constraints since the health service has always operated in the context of limited resources. The increasing involvement of doctors in management is not just a means for them to retain influence and power but it is sought by managers as well in order to increase organisational effectiveness in the quality of health care provided.

The research data suggests that potential benefits can accrue from managers and doctors working more closely together. This co-operation is dependent upon shared values which can be see to exist. Although there can be clear differences at individual levels these were not found along a simplistic dichotomy, for example, of managers being 'for' the reforms and clinicians being 'against'. The concept of managerialism and professionalism as companion processes is one that deserves further exploration. It is not the need for a management role that forms the basis for possible conflicts or inroads into professional power but the possibility that managers and professionals might have different priorities. Being at the 'sharp end', hospital doctors will feel the impact of reduced budgets more than their other colleagues in public health or general practice. In recognising that financial constraints were imposed from outside the unit, it proved possible in the case study sites for managers and professionals to agree shared objectives.

It is also necessary to recognise that the case study sites may not be representative of all units. Although professional autonomy at the operational level has generally been maintained, the growth in influence of the board at a strategic level where there is just one medical member and where two thirds of the non-executives come from the private sector, (Ashburner 1993a), must not be underestimated. This is where the major challenge to existing value systems is most likely to come from and the channel of communications falls very heavily onto a single person, the medical director.

The concept of autonomy can only be useful when integrated into a wider set of ideas about the relationship between professionals and managers, between professionals and organizations or between professionals and society. For the medical profession clinical autonomy can only be understood within an organizational and societal framework which can begin to produce a picture of how autonomy manifests itself and how it can and does change. Patterns of trade-offs between types of autonomy can be identified. For example, if part of a medical director's influence is due to their managerial position then such 'position power' might represent a broadening of criteria in the definition of their power base. This may represent a 'criteria too far' for theorists of the professions but many of the defining characteristics of the professions are shared by other expert groups that operate within an organizational setting and it therefore may be necessary to reassess the value of retaining professional groups as an entirely separate conceptual category.

The question has also been raised of whose autonomy? An important finding of this research was the significant changes that have occurred in the balance of power between different parts of the medical profession. This is important because it is difficult to argue that reductions in autonomy in one part of the profession denotes any lessening of total autonomy, when the cause is the increased power of other doctors. The shift in the balance of power between hospital doctors with GP fundholders and public health physicians has the potential to impact profoundly on the type and location of service provision, over which the hospital doctor has far less control than in the past.

Concluding comments

The roles of management and professionals can be seen as compatible but distinct despite the slight blurring of the boundary as represented by the involvement of some doctors in the management process. With the need for doctors to retain a predominantly clinical role if they are to have any credibility with their colleagues, there appears little prospect of many of them moving into purely management positions. This means that those doctors with a management role have the potential pressure that these possibly conflicting roles entail. What needs to be recognised is the way that structurally, responsibility has focused narrowly onto individual roles such as those of medical director and public health director. How these individuals continue to cope with their dual roles will be critical.

The lack of homogeneity within the profession and the clear examples of shifting power, suggest that there may be limits to the profession's ability to resist changes that might impinge on their autonomy, since many of these could be seen to be coming from within.

The process of change within the health service continues and there remains the potential for further challenges to the autonomy and power of the medical profession. Issues of audit and accountability continue, while those of junior doctors' hours, medical training and new European standards on the training requirements for the appointment of consultants, plus the Calman recommendations, will face hospital clinicians with further considerable challenges. GP fundholders still face the prospect of being cash limited and public health physicians still need to establish a firmer base for their speciality. In the search for economy, more managers are beginning to explore issues of skill mix which are also challenging professional boundaries.

The key to an understanding of the professions lies in seeing them in terms of relationships, within their profession, with other groups, with organizational settings and with work itself. An understanding of how susceptible a particular profession or occupational group is to challenges to its power base or autonomy lies in its ability to recognise the nature and significance of the changes facing it, and its willingness to adapt. Adaption, partly on their own terms, would appear more protective of their position in the long term than would imposition of change from outside.

References

Abbott, A. (1988), *The System of Professions: an essay on the division of expert labour,* University of Chicago Press, Chicago and London.

Ashburner, L. (1993a) 'The Composition of NHS Trust Boards: a national perspective' in Peck, E., Spurgeon, P. (eds.), *NHS Trusts in Practice*, Longman, Harlow.

Ashburner, L. (1993b) 'FHSAs: authorities in transition', Paper 8, *Authorities in the NHS*, NHSTD, Bristol.

Ashburner, L. and Cairncross, L. (1992), 'Members Attitudes and Expectations', Paper 5, *Authorities in the NHS*, NHSTD, Bristol.

Ashburner, L. and Cairncross, L. (1993), 'Membership of the 'new style' health authorities: continuity or change?', *Public Administration*, 71,3 357-375.

Ashburner, L., Ferlie, E. and FitzGerald, L. (1993), 'Boards and Authorities in Action', Paper 11, *Authorities in the NHS*, NHSTD, Bristol.

Ashburner, L., Ferlie, E. and Fitzgerald, L. (1995), 'Organisational transformation and top down change: the case of the NHS', *British Journal of Management*.

Atkinson, P. and Delamont, S. (1990), 'Professions and Powerlessness: female marginality in the learned occupations', *Sociological Review*, 38, 90-110.

Burns, T. (1981), 'A Comparative Study of Administrative Structure and Organisational Processes in Selected Areas of the NHS', *Research Report*, SSRC, London.

Cairncross, L., Ashburner L. and Pettigrew, A. (1991), 'Membership and Learning Needs', Paper 4, *Authorities in the NHS*, NHSTD, Bristol.

Calnan, M. and Gabe, J. (1991), 'Recent Developments in General Practice', in Gabe, J., Calnan, M. and Bury, M. (eds.) *The Sociology of the Health Service*, Routledge, London.

Cox, D. (1991), 'Health Service Management - a sociological view: Griffiths and the non-negotiated order of the hospital' in Gabe, J. et al. (eds), *The Sociology of the Health Service*, Routledge, London.

Davies, C. (1983), 'Professionals in Bureaucracies: the conflict thesis revisited' in Dingwall, R. and Lewis, P. (eds.) *The sociology of the professions: lawyers, doctors and others*, Macmillan, Basingstoke.

Department of Health (The Acheson Report), (1988), *Public Health in England*, HMSO, London.

Department of Health, (1989) *Working for Patients*, Cmnd. 555, HMSO, London.

Elcock, H. (1978), 'Regional government in action: the members of two RHAs' *Public Administration*, 56, 379-397.

Elston, M. A. (1991), 'The politics of professional power: medicine in a changing health service' in Gabe, J. et al, (eds.) *The Sociology of the Health Service*, Routledge, London.

Ferlie, E., FitzGerald, L. and Ashburner, L. (1992), 'The Challenge of Purchasing' Paper 7, *Authorities in the NHS*, NHSTD, Bristol.

FitzGerald, L. (1995), 'Clinicial management: the impact of a changing context on a changing profession', in Leopold, J., Glover, I. and Hughes, M. (eds), *Beyond Reason?*, Avebury, Aldershot.

Freidson, E. (1970), *Professional Dominance: the social structure of medical care*, Atherton Press, New York.

Freidson, E. (1986), 'The medical profession in transition' in Aiken, L. H. and Mechanic, D. (eds.) *Applications of Social Science to Clinical Medicine and Health Policy*, Rutgers University Press, New Brunswick.

Griffiths, R. (1983), *NHS Management Enquiry*, DHSS, London.

Hafferty, F. W. (1988), 'Theories at the Crossroads: a discussion of evolving views on medicine as a profession' *The Milbank Quarterly* 66, 2 202-225.

Hall, R. H. (1988), 'Comment on the sociology of the professions' *Work and Occupations*, 15, 273-275.

Halpern, S. A. (1992), 'Dynamics of professional control: internal coalitions and cross professional boundaries' *American Journal of Sociology*, 97, 994-1021.

Harrison, S. and Schultz, R. I. (1989), 'Clinical autonomy in the United Kingdom and the United States: contrasts and convergence' in Freddi, G. and Bjorkman, J. W. (eds), *Controlling Medical Professionals,* Sage, London.

Haug, M. R. (1973), 'Deprofessionalisation; an alternative hypothesis for the future' *Sociological Review Monograph* 20, 195-211.

Haug, M. R. (1988), 'A re-examination of the hypothesis of physician deprofessionalisation' *The Milbank Quarterly* 66, 2 48-56.

Kinston, W. (1983), 'Hospital organisation and structure and its effects on inter-professional behaviour and the delivery of care' *Social Science and Medicine* 17,16 1159-1170.

Klein, R. (1984), 'The politics of ideology versus the reality of politics: the case of Britain's NHS in the 1980s' *Milbank Memorial Fund Quarterly* 62, 82-108.

Larkin, G. (1988), 'Medical Dominance in Britain: image and historical reality' *The Milbank Quarterly* 66, 2 117-132.

Lemieux-Charles, L. (1992), 'Hospital-physician integration: case studies of community hospitals' *Health Services Management Research* 5,2 82-98.

McKinlay, J. B. (1988), 'Introduction' *The Milbank Quarterly* 66, 2 1-9.

McKinlay, J. B. and Arches, J. (1985), 'Towards the proletarianisation of physicians' *International Journal of Health Services* 15,2 161-195.

McKinlay, J. B. and Stoeckle, J. D. (1988), 'Corporatisation and the social transformation of doctoring' *International Journal of Health Services* 18,2 191-205.

Murray, T., Dingwall, R. and Eekelaar, J. (1983), 'Professionals in bureaucracies' in Dingwall, R. and Lewis, P. (eds), *The Sociology of the Professions: lawyers, doctors and others*, Macmillan, Basingstoke.

Navarro, V. (1988), 'Professional dominance or proletarianisation?: neither' *The Milbank Quarterly* 66,2 57-75.

Packwood, T., Keen J. and Buxton, M. (1992), 'Process and structure: resource management and the development of sub-unit organisational structure' *Health Services Management Research* 5,1 66-76.

Pritchard, P. (1987) 'Management development in primary health care', *Discussion paper*, Green College, Oxford.

Scott, W. R. (1985), 'Conflicting levels of rationality: regulators, managers and professionals in the medical care sector' *The Journal of Health Administration Education* 3,2 Pt II, 113-131.

Wolinsky, F.D. (1988), 'The professional dominance perspective revisited' *The Milbank Quarterly* 66,2 33-47.

12 Professions and management in the public sector: the experience of local government and the NHS in Britain

James Harrison and Sandra Nutley

Introduction

This chapter considers the relationship of professions and management in the public sector, particularly focusing on the National Health Service and local government in Britain. Both of these sub-sectors provide a rich setting within which to consider these issues. Both have historically been dominated by the professions (unlike, say, central government where the administrator has held greatest sway). Both have also been subject to ideological and structural changes from the 1970s onwards, with the express aim of introducing managerialism (Pollitt, 1990).

Although the rhetoric of managerialism in the public sector is by no means unique to Britain, the details of the changes occurring in this country can only be understood in the context of central government's desire to reduce publicexpenditure and withdraw the state from many aspects of life. Flynn (1990) has argued that the changes in approach to public service provision in Britain have been introduced in three main phases of getting expenditure under control, wearing down the opposition and introducing the market. Some of the measures introduced during each of these phases are summarised below:

Getting expenditure under control	Cash limits Value for money Market testing
Wearing down the opposition	Attack on the professions Decentralization Quality management and charters
Introducing the market	Split of policy and delivery Split of purchasers and providers Enabling not providing Internal markets

Hood (1991) argues that the changes occurring in the public sector amount to a new doctrine of public management. He goes on to highlight seven key elements of the doctrine: hands on professional management in the public sector; explicit standards and measures of performance; greater emphasis on output controls; shift to disaggregation of units in the public sector; shift to greater competition in the public sector; stress on private sector styles of management practice; stress on greater discipline and parsimony in resource use. Several commentators have warned us not to assume that the doctrine of managerialism is the reality of management within the public sector. Stewart and Walsh (1992) argue that in some cases the adoption of over-simplified private sector models has meant that the practical impact has been small. Olsen (1987, p. 3), writing about the Scandinavian experience has argued that: 'possibly private sector models have had more impact on how we talk about the public sector than on how it works.'

One element of the analysis of this chapter focuses on management/professions relations. The argument offered throughout the chapter is that there have been mixed messages as to the relationship between professionals and management. On the one hand, there have been seemingly clear messages about the need to involve professionals as managers of services (e.g. the Resource Management Initiative in the NHS as a means of involving clinicians in managerial decisions). On the other hand, there have been alternative messages about the need to impose management on professionals from outside (e.g. the initial idea was that General Manager appointments within the NHS would be 'professional managers' drawn from outside the main health service professions).

Another element of the analysis considers management/political relations. The paper looks at one of the more recent strategies for introducing managerialism into the public sector, that of appointing corporate style management boards consisting of a limited number of executive and non-executive board members (a reality for the newly styled health authorities, a one time proposal for police services and, at the time of writing, still a proposal for the Probation Service). This latest phase in the managerialist tradition is particularly interesting in that it brings into sharp focus the contradictions within the new public management ideology as enacted in Britain. For example, the newly styled, centrally appointed boards operate in stark contrast to notions of decentralization and greater local accountability (Stewart, 1993).

Before moving onto each of these themes the chapter first of all places the discussion in context by briefly considering what we mean by the terms professions and management and by reviewing some of the pertinent literature on the relationship between the two in the public sector. The paper then considers this relationship in the context of first the NHS and then local government. As domain theory (Kouzes and Mico, 1979) argues, there are three domains to consider in analysing public sector organisations: the professional, the managerial, and the political. For this reason the paper then goes onto consider the relationship of the political to the other two domains, particularly the managerial domain.

Professions, management and the public sector

Roach Anleu (1992, p. 23) comments that: 'much of the research and theorisation regarding the connection between the professions and bureaucratic administration has been to treat both of these categories as self-evident and homogeneous.' Looking first at the professions, much of the early (pre 1960s) research tried to reinforce this notion of homogeneity by considering the common attributes of those groups labelled as the professions. Millerson (1964) reviewed the work of 21 authors who tried to define the essential attributes of a true profession. He found 23 attributes which were regarded as essential, but no single attribute was accepted by all 21 authors. Roach Anleu (1992, p. 24) argues that:

> little consensus emerged on the irreducible attributes of a profession but those enumerated most frequently included: formal educational and entry requirements; a monopoly over an esoteric body of knowledge and associated skills; autonomy over the terms and conditions of practice; collegial authority; a code of ethics; and, a commitment to a service ideal.

Wilding (1982) points out that underlying the trait approach to the concept of the professions is an assumption of the functional role the professions. Carr-Saunders and Wilson (1964, p. 497) celebrated what they saw as the increasing importance of the profession as the 'stabilising elements in society' and Parsons (1937, 1951) likewise emphasised the functionality of the professions. Since the 1960s the trait approach to defining a profession has given way to one which considers the concept of the professions in terms of occupational control. This enables us to consider the way in which certain occupational groups have established power over other groups, the public and their clients (Freidson, 1970; Johnson, 1972).

Distinctions are made between different types of profession. Morgan (1990) distinguishes between, on the one hand, doctors, lawyers and accountants and, on the other, teachers and social workers. The former are said to have been founded on the basis of serving well-off individuals who voluntarily sought professional help. The latter have their foundation in being employed by the state to work with an involuntary clientele. Carr-Saunders and Wilson (1964) distinguished between the established professions and the semi-professions. The former are said to be based upon the theoretical study of a particular area and prescribed norms of behaviour. Whilst the latter replace theoretical study by the acquisition of technical skills. Hearn (1982) notes that there is an inter-relationship between patriarchy and professionalisation. The established professions being dominated by men, the semi-professions being the domain of women.

Management is no more homogeneous a concept than that of the professions. The variety of managerial work and the diversity of those who have the title of 'manager' is summarised by Torrington, Weightman and Johns (1989). Writers commenting upon the concept of management being employed in the private sector stress its emphasis upon rationality and its domination by financial calculation and accountability (Child et al., 1983; Spybey, 1984).

The relationship between management and the professions has a rich history of inquiry. The debate is multifaceted because it encompasses: the existence of the professions within management (Child et al., 1983); the professionalisation of management (Reed and Anthony, 1992); and the extent to which the professions are controlled by management or vice-versa (Raelin, 1985). As the introduction to this chapter points out, the form of managerialism which has been introduced into the public sector over recent years stresses rationality and calculation. "The dominance of calculability and rationalisation in private sector firms provide a powerful model of legitimacy which undermines abstract notions of 'service' or 'the public good'" (Morgan, 1990, p. 124).

One of the features of the new public management doctrine is the adoption of private sector management styles and organizational forms. This can be related to the notion of institutional isomorphism developed by DiMaggio and Powell (1983), where isomorphism is a 'constraining process that forces one unit of a population to resemble other units that face the same set of environmental conditions'. DiMaggio and Powell (1983, p. 150) identify three mechanisms of institutional isomorphic change:

1   coercive isomorphism that stems from political influence and the problem of legitimacy;

2   mimetic isomorphism resulting from standard responses to uncertainty; and

3   normative isomorphism, associated with professionalization.

All three mechanisms can be identified as operating in the public sector, as the case studies of the NHS and local government below demonstrate. Morgan (1990) argues that normative isomorphism has been particularly important in the past. Greenwood and Stewart (1986) have likewise noted the importance of professional networks in diffusing the fashionable solutions to organizational problems. In the present context of the new public management, Morgan notes that there has been a colonisation of the public sector by private sector professionals, particularly accountants, and that this is leading to a new form of normative isomorphism. However, as pointed out above, we need to be cautious about accepting the rhetoric of the new public management at face value. Morgan argues that there is a gap between the myth of institutional isomorphism and the actual situation in these organisations. This gap is said to derive from two features:

1   the power-knowledge dialectic which is a dynamic process of resistance and non-compliance;

2   alternative bases of organization legitimation - rationality and calculation are only one basis of legitimation, others include citizenship and equality.

In the public sector the relationship between professionals and administration/management has frequently been depicted as one of conflict. There is a swath of research which stresses the incompatibility of bureaucratic and professional norms (Barber, 1963; Merton, 1968; Hall, 1972). Domain theory is built upon the premise of this conflict, but argues that there are more than two parties involved. Kouzes and Mico (1979) argue that in order to understand behaviour in, what they term, Human Service Organizations we need to consider the interaction between three distinct domains - policy, management and service. They theorise that each domain gives rise to its own legitimacy norms which contrast with the norms of the other.

The result of the interaction of these domains is an organization that is internally disjunctive and discordant. The three domains are characterised as follows (Kouzes and Mico, 1979, p. 458):

	Policy	Management	Service
Principles	Consent of the governed	Hierarchical Control & coordination	Autonomy Self-regulation
Success Measures	Equity	Cost efficiency Effectiveness	Quality of service Good standards of practice
Structure	Representative Participation	Bureaucratic	Collegial
Work modes	Voting Bargaining Negotiation	Use of linear techniques & tools	Client-specific Problem-solving
People/ actors	Elected officials	Managers	Service deliverers

The emphasis upon conflict between professionals and management is in danger of being overemphasized. Roach Anleu (1992, p. 23) argues, based upon her research on social workers, that the relationship is more one of dependence:

> conflict and tension arising from specific bureaucratic requirements combined with professional workers' claims for autonomy are not the invariable or inevitable outcome of organisational employment. Indeed, by defining spheres

231

of competence and exclusive jurisdiction, organisational guide-lines protect social workers from encroachment by, and competition with members of other professions....In addition, social workers depend upon complex organisations for essential resources including employment opportunities and clients thereby contributing to professional- organisational interdependence and integration.

The argument about the inevitable conflict between professionals and the rationalizing tendencies of management are also countered by Morgan (1990, p. 124) who points out that:

although these same professions may in certain respects dislike and resist the implications of rationality, their general commitment to expertise makes a wholesale opposition to rationalization impossible.

Research by Green (1975) has pointed out that conflict in a group of Scottish hospitals was not so much between doctors and administrators, but rather between sub-groups of professionals. Similarly, Strauss et al. (1963) considered the negotiated order within hospitals and the importance of inter professional negotiation. Houlihan (1988) argues that the 1980s proved to be a hostile period for the professions within the public sector. He identifies a number of sources of this increased hostility:

1 a shift away from a commitment to welfare state collectivism - the ideology of professionalism being best suited to notions of the welfare state;

2 increased standards of education and a growing middle class which has led to an increasing willingness to challenge professional judgements;

3 the emergence of a new breed of elected member who is less deferential and more sceptical of professional advice;

4 evidence of professional failure - high rise flats, urban motorways, town centre redevelopments (Gyford, 1984).

Houlihan adds that the challenges are not only external, there are, he says, clear signs of increasing self doubt among many public sector professionals.

The NHS: a suitable case for treatment

The pattern of reform

The themes of the new public management described in the introduction are easily discernible in the series of initiatives to which the NHS was subject throughout the

1980s and early 1990s. Initial measures were directed to making the then system more effective; for example, the Rayner Scrutinies in 1982 and the advent of performance indicators in 1983, both to the accompaniment of a more general concern with the efficient use of land, labour and capital. These eventually gave way to a qualitatively quite different set of strategies which sought much more profound change: the community care initiatives (DHSS, 1986; DHSS, 1989a) designed to change fundamentally the pattern of service delivery; the nation wide health targets (DoH, 1991a) which promulgate explicit outcomes; quality (DHSS 1989b) and charter initiatives (DoH, 1991b) which reinforce a customer-centred orientation. Arguably, however, of such substantial strategies, the two most important were the introduction of General Management and, more recently, the implementation of the *Working for Patients* (DHSS, 1989b) reforms. The culture change which is said to have resulted from this programme of change are summarised in Figure 12.1

From:	To:
Centralised control	Decentralised decision making
Concern for procedures	Concern for outputs
Preoccupation with operations	Concern for customers
Functional specialization	Cross-functional working
Rules	Values
Cost	Price

Figure 12.1   Culture change in the NHS

Source: *Adapted from NHSTD, 1991, p. 3*

Any attempt to understand management/professional relations must take place against the policy backdrop of what was intended and an appreciation of what actually happened. Described below is a case study of the implementation of General Management in a single English District Health Authority (DHA) as a vehicle to illuminate the early effects of reform upon management/professional relations in the NHS.

The introduction of general management in the NHS - a case study

The Management Inquiry was set up by the Rt Hon Norman Fowler, the then Secretary of State for Health & Social Security:

> to review current initiatives to improve the efficiency of the health service in England and to advise on the management action needed to secure the best value for money and the best possible service to patients (Fowler, 1983).

The findings were set out in a letter to the Secretary of State which was published in June 1983, subsequently to become widely known as the Griffiths Report (DHSS, 1983). The report advocated a number of radical developments which included change within the DHSS itself, greater prominence for the personnel and property function(s) and, despite streamlining consultation procedures, a consumerist emphasis. The most radical proposal, however, was to be the introduction of general management in place of functional management. This was defined as, 'the responsibility drawn together in one person at different levels of the organisation for planning, implementation and control of performance (Fowler, 1983, p. 11).' Despite a vigourous debate and the active resistance of the professions the report's recommendations were fully implemented throughout the NHS.

The second half of the report set out some of the reasoning behind the recommendations: individual overall management accountability could not be located; the machinery of implementation was generally weak; a lack of orientation towards performance in the service; a lack of concern with the views of consumers of health services. This was a picture consistent with a subsequent analysis which concluded that the NHS, between 1960-82, was not a unitary organisation, was dominated by the professions (particularly medicine), where change was incremental/marginal and in which the management culture was that of diplomacy where managers acted as maintainers (Harrison et al., 1989a).

The research reported here began in 1988, five years after the Griffiths Report. At that time there had been relatively few attempts to evaluate the impact of General Management. A variety of authors identified critical prerequisites (e.g. Dearden, 1985; Stewart & Smith, 1988); others brought a practitioner perspective (e.g. Barbour, 1989; Wall, 1989; Nicholls, 1989); a few sought to explore differing outcomes (e.g. Alleway, 1987; Strong & Robinson, 1990). The most comprehensive evaluation, however, was that of Harrison et al. (1989a and b; 1991). They concluded that although progress had been made in respect of changes in formal organization structure, the allocation of personal responsibility, speed of decision making and performance management, substantial difficulties remained with consumer responsiveness and with management budgeting/resources management. In this context, their comment that 'the deepest shadows... cloak the relations between general managers and the medical profession' (Harrison et al., 1989a, p.16) was a telling observation.

The research site for the case study reported here was a single urban District Health Authority (DHA) serving a population of 240,000 with a budget of £54 million. The study was carried out in two phases: participant observation and documentary analysis in 1988-89 and a systematic postal survey of the 49 most senior managers during 1989-90. The survey population consisted of all the members of the District Management Board, each Unit Management Team together with director, nurse manager and administrator in each of the ten Programmes. The response rate was 97.9 per cent. The findings have been fully detailed elsewhere (Harrison & Nutley, 1993) and therefore only broad themes will be considered.

The implementation of general management can be thought of as having three elements: infrastructure, systems and a concern with a corporate or strategic focus. The data in both phases of the research were collected and can be reported in a manner consistent with such a framework. Infrastructure tended to be the most visible and widely supported element of implementation. The number of Units reduced from five to three but was accompanied by the birth of ten 'Programmes' centred upon clinical specialty or client group which 'cut across' Unit structure. This was accompanied by substantial changes to functional management, with staff in a number of disciplines ceasing to report to senior professionals in a strictly functional hierarchy, in favour of less senior professionals or non professionals in a Unit setting. These developments took place against a backdrop of increasing tension as the interests of the District and the Units diverged, and as the disadvantages of the matrix structure made themselves felt (Davis & Lawrence, 1988). Clinical professionals became increasingly unhappy with the general pattern of change and with a sense of dispossession.

The development of the relevant management systems was the area of greatest difficulty. The establishment of a performance management directorate was an innovative development but this was in marked contrast to disappointing progress in respect of decision making and very poor performance in respect of financial systems. Decision making proved to be speedier and more effective in operational settings than in the strategic domain. Financial systems were poorly developed and only partially aligned with the complex organizational structure. The combination of poor strategic decision making and inadequate financial systems proved to be a potent cocktail and contributed significantly to the District's subsequent financial crisis.

In terms of the corporate/strategic focus, performance here was heavily and negatively influenced by poor strategic decision making. This, however, was compounded by little or no attention being given to the development of the personnel and property function(s) as had been advocated in the original Griffiths Report findings. The former did eventually receive attention, in the form of scrutiny and development. The Estates function did not play the strategically critical role anticipated by Griffiths, and was effectively marginalised. Progress with customer relations was good, if a little one sided. The DHA developed a formidable capacity to communicate information to its local community but was perhaps less effective in listening and responding to its wishes.

As a post script to the study, the DHA merged with its neighbour in 1991 on the same day that the WfP reforms were introduced. This ultimately had the effect of changing the number and nature of Units again and the Programme structure effectively disappeared in due course. The financial difficulties matured into a £30 million deficit and the resultant crisis ultimately prompted the departure of the Director of Finance, the Chairman and the CEO.

Discussion

Overall staff in the district viewed the introduction of general management in a positive way. The exceptions were their views of the impact of management budgets and resource management. This picture is not too dissimilar from that found by Harrison et al. (1989a). Positive perceptions of outcomes were not, however, evenly distributed. The District Headquarters was the most positive, the Acute Unit the least, particularly regarding the Programme Director role and the contribution of professionals. Any consideration of the Programme Director role has to appreciate that of the ten posts, eight were occupied by clinicians, of which five were doctors. Whilst clinicians were involved in management, the nature of that involvement was more apparent than real. With regard to the doctors occupying Programme Director posts: their accountability to general management was in terms of their part-time management role rather than as a clinician; their role with regard to their respective programmes was one of providing 'programme leadership' together with 'clinical integrity and direction' rather than exercising conventional management control; whatever the precise definition, the authority they exercised - particularly with regard to their peers - was by consent.

It is difficult to deny the conclusion that 'most doctors and most managers continue to inhabit a shared culture of medical autonomy' (Harrison et al., 1989b, p. 44). Other professional groups (e.g. nursing and estates) fared less well. This was exemplified by the view they expressed in the postal survey, in which they were markedly less positive in their view of general management than other respondents. In conclusion, the advent of general management: challenged the authority of the professionals by questioning practice; denied the moral supremacy claimed by professionals by substituting quality for ethics; weakened professional identity and coherence by encouraging cross functional working/revised structural arrangements; made professionals more transparent and therefore accessible as a result of flatter organisations and the 'death' of middle management (Harrison & Thompson, 1992). Although such forces have reduced the power and influence of professional groups, general management has had only limited success in harnessing and directing the more senior profession of medicine. These professionals continue to act as a restraining influence upon management. For this reason the most powerful groups are courted, the least are not, and both are increasingly to be found in the domain of the clinical directorate.

236

Whether the WfP reforms will have greater impact in the longer term remains to be seen. Dent (1993, p. 265) is of the opinion that there is already evidence of such an impact:

> Whether the re-organisation of the NHS leads to the improvement or decline in the quality of care the changes do involve a fundamental change in the relationship between doctors and the state. Doctors have conceded that clinical autonomy is now subject to resource constraints.... In principle the new organisational arrangement involve the medical profession accepting the principles of *responsible autonomy* within an overall system of managerial control. (original emphasis).

Local government: the quiet revolution?

The pattern of reform

Stewart (1990) has described the years 1945-75 as ones of relative stability. The growing need for service was so clear; there was a right solution to most of the problems - all that was needed was an increased capacity to deliver them. Since 1975 uncertainty and discontinuity are frequently taken as more apt descriptions of life in local government. Although whether this amounts to a 'revolution in progress' (Major, 1989, p. 1) still remains to be seen.

Stewart and Walsh (1992) highlight three main areas of legislative reform in local government in England and Wales during the above latter period:

1 compulsory competitive tendering (in 1980 and 1988) requiring local authorities to put out to tender a specified range of services;

2 the Education Reform Act (1988) introducing changes which include the national curriculum, national assessment tests, the local management of schools, and the ability for schools to opt out of local authority control;

3 community care (1990) whereby local authorities are to become assessors of local need and the purchasers of services to meet this need from a range of providers.

Stewart and Walsh note, however, that legislation is not the only trigger for change in local government. Individual local authorities have also shaped their own agenda with regards to areas such as performance measurement and management, competition, the introduction of internal trading units, decentralization and flexible pay and conditions.

The period since 1974 has seen a number of changes in the prevalent ideology of local government. Following the 1974 reorganisation of local government and the issuing of the Bains Report (1972), the ideology of corporate management dominated the 1970s. By the beginning of the 1980s, corporate management as an ideology was beginning to wane. Cuts in central government support were biting more deeply and unemployment was rising. Despite the continuing rhetoric of corporatism, departmentalism was strong. The 1980s saw the rise of a new ideology and a set of structures to go with it. The ideology was consumerism and the associated structures were those of decentralized service delivery and managerial responsibility. There had been an assumption that local authorities provide as well as organize and administer services. This assumption of self-sufficiency came under attack during the 1980s, with the development of new visions of local authorities as The Competitive Council (Audit Commission, 1988), or The Enabling Council (Clark and Stewart, 1988).

Professionalism has been considered as a defining feature of local government (Houlihan, 1988), but this has not shielded these professions from criticism. Poole (1978, p. 44) has been one of the most outspoken critics:

> ...segregation of professionals into separate departments each supervised by a committee (leading) allegedly, to services ... promoted to gratify professional aspirations rather than to meet the needs of the community as a whole.

The reforms of the 1980s can be seen as a direct challenge to local government professionalism. Stewart and Walsh (1992) argue that whilst some of the challenges (particularly to excessive professional autonomy) are seen as welcome, there are some issues which remain to be faced:

> Thus, while it can be argued that in certain parts of the public sector, the professional culture was over-dominant, that does not mean that the professional role is not important. Or while it can be argued that traditional modes of accountability prevented responsiveness to the customer, that does not mean that public service can be totally responsive to the customer or that political accountability should be disregarded. (Stewart and Walsh, 1992, p. 511).

Houlihan (1988, p. 73) argues that there are tentative signs that some local government professionals are beginning to 'outgrow the need for a professional shield to protect their occupation and that some may even find professionalism inhibiting'. This is especially so, it is argued, as senior staff in local government try to fit new interests and tasks into existing patterns of professional departments and expertise. Interestingly, though, these comments are made in a paper which focuses on one 'junior' service (Leisure Services) trying to obtain professional status.

The implementation of change in local government - a case study

The case study site is a metropolitan district council in England. It covers an area of almost 38 square miles and had a resident population of approximately 300,000 in 1987. At this time the council employed nearly 13,000 staff within 12 departments and had a revenue budget of some £150 million. This made it one of the larger metropolitan district councils, with one of the smallest ratios of staff per head of population. The data for this case study was collected over the period 1985-87, data was collected from documentary sources, interviews and questionnaires. The detailed case study is presented elsewhere (Nutley, 1991). What follows is a brief summary of some of the main themes, which can be used to inform the professions and management debate. The newly amalgamated borough council started off in 1974, in the words of one interviewee, as 'full of enthusiasm and high hopes'. Budgets were expanding and client groups were growing. These early years were a time when corporate working was given a high priority. There was soon a set-back to this enthusiasm as the problems of financial constraint hit the authority. There followed from the mid 1970s onwards a constant battle to cut back expenditure in the face of growing demands for certain services. Although there were changes in the 1970s - changes in political control, an end to service expansion and some experiments with new forms of organisation and service delivery - the 1970s were characterised by relative continuity in terms of the main actors and organisational structure. By contrast, the 1980s witnessed greater uncertainty in relation to political control, the acceleration of environmental changes (e.g. unemployment), major reviews of departmental and corporate structures, and a sharp increase in the turnover of senior officers. The deteriorating economic situation and the rise in levels of unemployment was associated with economic issues taking a higher profile in the council. The 1980s also brought the beginnings of competition. In addition to implementing legislation, the council voluntarily went out to tender for school's cleaning in 1982. By the early 1980s the discussion in committees and memos was about improving efficiency, cutting costs and regenerating the local economy. The slogans of corporatism had been replaced with those of value for money.

In addition to the changes at the council wide level, developments were taking place in individual service departments. For example, the further education sphere was becoming increasingly competitive, with the local authority having to bid for funds. The traditional independence of local authority education was declining with the introduction of the Manpower Services Commission as a new source of funding and policy development. In the Public Works Department the fleet management unit (not at that time effected by legislation) began to operate along commercial lines. The attitude of the engineers in this department was very positive:

We are technical people who have been working with the private sector all our lives. Most of us welcomed the changes, those who didn't have gone and those who were pro-change have risen to the top (Public Works Manager).

Discussion

It is tempting to try and personify the professions and management by identifying those who are primarily professionals and those who are managers. This is not possible in the case study in question because virtually all middle and senior staff had the credentials of a professional association and were working in the service delivery area of that profession. The main exceptions are those (few in number) who were working in the Chief Executive's office. As pointed out in the previous section, the case study authority was not unique in this way. Poole (1978) suggests that professional dominance of senior positions is a primary characteristic of local government service. The conflict within this authority can not be characterised as conflict between professionals and generic managers. The question which remains to be answered is whether the conflict was one of professionalism versus managerialism. Departmental interests were one of the main shaping forces throughout the period studied. There were several examples of changes being tamed by departmentalism. Attempts to introduce a more rational process into budgetary planning were said to have been re-shaped by chief officers and their chairs of committee working together to protect departmental interests. However, departmental interests do not directly equate with professional interests, nor do they necessarily conflict with the new managerialism. It would be more accurate to say that departmental senior managers quickly embraced many tenets of the new managerialism (like performance measurement, decentralization, and competition) as a means of taming any threat such initiatives may have imposed, by interpreting them and implementing them within the context of the interests of their own departments.

Wilding (1982) outlines the nature and extent of professional power within the welfare state under five headings: power in policy making and administration; power to define needs and problems; power in resource allocation; power over people; power to control the area of work. It is clear in the case study site that departmental chief officers (often in conjunction with their elected committee chairs) used the doctrine of the new managerialism in such a way as to ensure that they lost little in relation to each of the above areas of power. The conflict within the authority tended to be interdepartmental and between professions rather than between professionalism and managerialism. Managerialism was used in this rivalry as part of the battle to secure at least level funding and to maintain a separate departmental existence. However, it would be wrong to suggest that senior managers whole-heartedly adopted the accounting rationalization and calculation of the managerial doctrine. They learnt the language and then proceeded to use it to their advantage. The divergence between managerialism and professionalism tended to be felt more at the front line level of social workers and teachers. These individuals were increasingly subject to reduced autonomy and a need to justify their actions and document their performance.

Overall, though, the argument being developed here (which is in line with that of Roach Anleu, 1992) is that organizational procedures and managerialist approaches can act to protect professional groups from encroachment by other professional groups. Important aspects of department status and the status quo were protected by 'modernising' from within.

The political domain and management/professional relations

The conventional distinction drawn between politics and administration is rooted in a system of checks and balances, in which the executive draws its legitimacy from elected individuals within a democratic framework. This is an approach which produces salaried, professionally trained career officials and elected transitory amateurs. The work of Weber (1919) explores this differentiation of the polity which Derlien (1988, p. 132) summarises in the following terms:

> politicians cope with what may be called *normative complexity*, while the function of civil servants can be seen as reducing *factual uncertainty* by relying on routines and applying professional expertise... only politicians are in a position to bring about *substantive rationality*, whereas civil servants produce at best *formal rationality*. (Original emphasis)

In short there is supposedly an ends-means and values-facts dichotomy. Politicians allocate the values, civil servants bring expression to them. As noted in the introduction, the advent of managerialist strategies (Pollitt, 1990) throughout the 1980s and 90s has seen public administration evolve into 'public management' (Gunn, 1988) within the wider context of the 'new public management' (Hood, 1991). This has inevitably had consequences for all the major actors - politicians, managers and professionals - which some commentators have sought to understand with the use of domain theory (e.g. Edmonstone, 1986).

The view expressed by Stewart & Walsh (1992) is that a feature of public sector reform is the attempt to separate the political process from the management process. This is in line with the managerialist doctrine which argues that 'managers should be free to manage' The DoE (1991) consultation paper on the internal management of local authorities set out a number of alternative futures for management/ political relations, but with the clear message of the need for a clearer definition and distinction of roles. Leach et al. (1992) argue that in local government the role of elected members, with regard to service provision, has been reduced, both as a result of legislation (CCT) and as a result of pressure from groups such as the Audit Commission. The latter advocate the withdrawal of member involvement in 'detail'. Stewart and Walsh note, however, that practice may differ from intention. The argument in this paper is that in the NHS, in particular, intention and reality do appear to be at odds.

In the NHS, one might point to a gap between the political role of the Secretary of State and the management role of the NHS Management Board, as it was formally, to illustrate the separation of politics and management. However, the resignation of Victor Page, its first chairman, allegedly over his right to manage, suggests that political necessity far outweighed political rhetoric. Another example of the same phenomenon was the frequent interventions of the then Secretary of State, Kenneth Clarke, during the course of the long running Ambulance Service dispute.

Any critique of the reformed NHS would almost certainly identify the appointment of RHA/DHA/FHSA/NHS Trust Chairmen/women - by the Secretary of State - as political appointments. The appointment of Robin Buchanan to Wessex RHA and Sir Donald Wilson, on an interim basis, to the West Midlands RHA, are clear examples of the political appointment of business men to manage particularly troubled areas. The same is true, if somewhat less obvious, of HA, FHSA and NHS Trust chairs. In key settings, the local chair is now only a phone call away from the Secretary of State. This proximity and interdependence can bring its own honours and rewards, or, when things go wrong, disapprobation.

The new HAs and NHS Trust boards are required to operate on a more business-like basis. Indeed, they mimic the composition and operation of private sector boards. In the end the lay politician becomes almost indistinguishable from the executives. The issue is not that such matters are unworthy of their detailed attention, but that the distinctiveness of separate role and function all but disappears. In this regard the Cadbury Report (1992), which warns of the dangers of combining the role of chair/CEO and reinforces the need for prudent corporate governance, is a timely reminder.

Whilst it is argued that politicians have journeyed to the managerial domain, it is also contended that managers have and continue to travel in the opposite direction. An important early phase in this process is, perhaps, the emergence of so called 'visionary leadership' as the model for NHS managers. Duncan Nichol (1990) said of it:

> Leaders... are people who positively and proactively assert their personal convictions in addition to the values and purposes of their organisation and do so in a way that excites others and inspires them to follow.

Whilst careful not to make more of the point than it warrants, this appears to go beyond the assumption that officials will exercise discretion and human judgement in the implementation of policy (Lipsky, 1980). Rather, it implies that this is now an explicit requirement and as a consequence, policy is shaped - at least in part - by overt executive aspiration and preference.

It is precisely because of their familiarity with and understanding of health policy and management that senior managers either seek or are invited to contribute to the higher levels of the policy forming process. Vertical integration is aided by the 'free movement of labour' which takes place between the Service and the DOH and/or the NHS Management Executive (and vice versa). Equally important is the movement between the Service and a growing number of specialist academic centres/think tanks which themselves may be associated with the centre and policy formation. In this way the gap between managers and politicians or more accurately between management and the political process narrows.

In the end state it may be difficult for the observer or the observed to be absolutely sure whether a manager is in the managerial or the political domain. This is most readily observed, but not universally so, in the reformed HAs and NHS Trusts, in which executive and non executive members enjoy equal corporate status. Whilst it is true that executives have specialist managerial roles, in corporate format they have to fulfil the duties and obligations required of any member of a public authority. The policy of the organization is explicitly shaped by their contribution, the choices to be made in allocating scarce resources is influenced by their preferences, the extent to which the authority displays responsibility, integrity and rectitude is a function of the moral climate of which they are a part. These are not only or simply facets of the managerial repertoire, they are fundamentally concerned with the allocation of values and are therefore political in character.

This section has sought to explore the managerial/political interface. It has rejected the view that in the NHS, in particular, public sector reform has resulted in the separation of the political from the management process. An alternative view is advanced which argues that reform has progressively drawn politicians into the management domain and managers into the political domain. The resultant milieu has a number of consequences for the actors and for society: the gap between managers and politicians has closed considerably and therefore the normal checks and balances have been weakened; the increase in the number of political appointees has reduced accountability; politicians or political appointees have short time horizons and may therefore may be inclined to expediency and be overly concerned with matters of presentation; senior managers are increasingly becoming personalities; fixed term contracts and appraisal systems encourage short term horizons and, coupled with the above, can lead to impression management; senior managers working in a political environment become pragmatic about what is acceptable rather than what is right.

Trends such as these raise important questions of accountability and performance. This is all the more important as managers and politicians converge in the common pursuit of success and the avoidance of failure. Whether similar outcomes will be experienced in local government remains to be seen. Leach et al. (1992) report that the management/political distinction at present is wrought with confusion and uncertainty. The impact is more likely to be felt at the service level as local government increasingly splinters into ever more independent services. The experience of school governing bodies and the newly styled 'probation boards' (which still await the enabling legislation) will be instructive. But what does all this mean for management / professional relationships? This question is addressed in the concluding section of this paper.

Conclusions

One of the main conclusions to be drawn from the research and discussion presented in this paper is that it would be inadvisable to treat the public sector in a cursory and over generalised way when considering the professions and management. Taking the NHS and local government as two examples, the reforms of the 1980s appear to have effected them both in different ways.

In the NHS there were the beginnings of a relatively clear separation of management and professional tasks with the establishment of general managers. This has subsequently been reinforced by a growing coalition between managers and politicians within the newly styled authorities and boards established at various levels within the NHS. There has been a decline in professional power, particularly with regards to Wilding's (1982) categories of policy making, defining needs and resource allocation. Such a decline in professional power is not so evident with regard to control over people and areas of work.

In local government, there is not, as yet, a clearly identifiable management cadre. Managerial tasks and approaches have been colonised by professional bodies and incorporated as part of their professional practice. Unlike the NHS, where the most recent alliance appears to be between the managerial and political domains, in local government the professional and political domains continue to provide a powerful alliance in shaping local policies and practices. Although commentators (such as Houlihan, 1988) point to the hostile environment for local government professionals and internal self doubt, there is, as yet, little concrete evidence of reduced power. Indeed some of the reforms can be said to have strengthened the hand of certain professionals (e.g. social workers) and in other areas (such as teaching) the professions have shown a remarkable ability to resist many overt challenges to their occupational control. The introduction of National Standards, performance measurement and external reporting can all be seen as important challenges to the professions. However, it is important to remember that these initiatives are being implemented by the professionals themselves and often in ways which continue to preserve their own positions. Things may change if the internal management of local authority reviews lead to the creation of council managers and cabinet style government.

The above two pen pictures of the NHS and local government conceal as much as they reveal. As Carr-Saunders and Wilson (1964) and Morgan (1990) point out, it may be instructive to look at differences in terms of the established versus the semi-professions. It is also useful to consider differences within professional groups, particularly between the more senior and junior members.

In the NHS it is clear that the established medical profession have lost least in terms of occupational control and organizational power. This is in contrast to the more semi-profession of nursing. In both the NHS and local government the front line professionals have been the ones who have suffered the most. Senior professionals have had the opportunity and/ or ability to adopt the changes and align themselves with the dominant coalition. The front-line professionals have generally felt the most challenged, scrutinised, oppressed and marginalised.

The generalised sense of malaise that pervades the public sector can be explained on the grounds of a sense of loss, a mourning for an earlier golden age. It can also be seen as a legitimate concern about problematic goals, strategies and outcomes (e.g. specific concerns by managers about what professionals should do and by professionals about how managers conduct themselves - ends and means).

The received wisdom that any attempt to restrain professional aspirations inevitably results in conflict between managers and professionals is not universally true. A new pragmatism - perhaps born out of a decade of public sector reform, coupled with recession and high levels of unemployment - suggests that there are few 'no go' areas. Members of challenged professional groups negotiate. They no longer do this entirely via the representations of their professional bodies. As the reforms have progressed the relationship between individual professionals and their employing organizations appears to have changed. Prior to the reforms, these individuals appeared to primarily identify with their professional group, their membership of the employing organization was secondary. As the reforms progressed there appeared to be a shift (in the NHS, at least) towards identifying with the corporate organization first and foremost. More recently identification with the corporate organization appears to be collapsing as individuals are increasingly encouraged to negotiate their own employment terms and conditions. This seems to lead individuals to focus much more narrowly on their own individual contracts and requirements. Such an individual focus may bring positive benefits in terms of increased flexibility and the breakdown of increasingly artificial professional barriers (which Normand, 1993, argues for in the case of the NHS). However, there may well be problems in reconciling such self interest *en masse* with the requirements of the public interest.

References

Alleway, L. (1987), 'Back on the outside looking in', *The Health Service Journal* 16th July: 818-819.

Audit Commission (1988), *The Competitive Council*, London: HMSO.

Bains, M. (1972), *The New Local Authorities: Management and Structure*, London: HMSO.

Barber, B. (1963), 'Some problems in the sociology of the professions', *Daedulus* 92: 669-688.

Barbour, J. (1989) 'Notions of "success" in general management', *Health Services Management Research* 2(1): 53-57.

Cadbury, A. (1992), *Report of the committee on the financial aspects of corporate governance in the UK*, London.

Carr-Sanders, A. M. and Wilson, P. A. (1964), *The Professions*, London: Frank Cass.

Child, J., Fores, M., Glover, I. & Lawrence, P. (1983), 'A price to pay? professionalism and work organisation in Britain and West Germany', *Sociology*, 17: 63-77.

Clarke, M. & Stewart, J. (1988), *The Enabling Council*, Luton: Local Government Training Board.

Davis, S. M. & Lawrence, P. R. (1988), *Matrix*, London: Addison-Wesley.

Dearden, R. W. (1985), 'The development of general management', *Hospital and Health Service Review*, July: 163-164.

Dent, M. (1993), 'Professionalism, educated labour and the state: hospital medicine and the new managerialism', *The Sociological Review*, 41: 244-273.

Derlien, H-U. (1988), 'Public managers and politics' in Kooiman, J. & Eliassen, K. A., *Managing Public Organizations*, London, Sage.

DiMaggio, P. J. & Powell, W. W. (1983), 'The iron cage revisited: institutional isomorphism and collective rationality in organisational fields', *American Sociological Review*, 48: 147-160.

DoE (1991, *The internal management of local authorities in England*: a consultation paper, London, Department of the Environment.

DHSS (1983), *NHS Management Inquiry* (Griffiths Report), London, HMSO.

DHSS (1986), *Neighbourhood nursing: a focus for care* (The Cumberlege Report), London, HMSO.

DHSS (1989a), *Caring for people - community care in the next decade and beyond*, London, HMSO.

DHSS (1989b), *Working for Patients* (white paper), London, HMSO.

DoH (1991a), *The health of the nation*, London, HMSO.

DoH (1991b), *The Patients Charter*, London, HMSO.

Edmonstone, J. D. (1986), 'If you're not the woodcutter, what are you doing with the axe?', *Health Services Manpower Review*, 12(3): 8-12.

Fowler, N. (1983), *Statement on the NHS inquiry*, 26th October, London, Department of Health & Social Security.

Flynn, N. (1990), *Public Sector Management*, London: Harvester Wheatsheaf.

Freidson, E. (1970), Professional dominance: the social structure of medical care, New York: Atherton.

Green, S. (1975), 'Professional/bureaucratic conflict; the case of the medical profession in the NHS', *The Sociological Review*, 23: 121-138.

Greenwood, R. & Stewart, J. (1986), 'The institutional and organisational capabilities of local government', *Public Administration*, 64: 35-50.

Gunn, L. (1988), 'Public management: a third approach', *Public Money and Management* 8 (1&2): 21-25.

Gyford, J. (1984), *Local Politics in Britain*, London, Croom Helm.

Hall, R. H. (1972), 'Professionalisation and bureaucratisation' in Pavalko, R. M. (ed.), *Sociological Perspectives on Occupations*, F. E. Peacock.

Harrison, J. and Nutley, S. (1993), 'Whither health service management?', in Malek, M., Vacani, P., Rasquinha, J. & Davey, P. (eds), *Managerial Issues in the Reformed NHS*, Chicester, Wiley.

Harrison, J. & Thompson, D. (1992), 'A flat earth syndrome', *Health Service Journal*, 17th September: 29.

Harrison, S., Hunter, D. J., Marnoch, G. & Pollitt, C. (1989a), *General management in the NHS: before and after the White Paper*, Leeds, Nuffield Institute.

Harrison, S., Hunter, D. J., Marnoch, G. & Pollitt, C. (1989b), 'General management and medical autonomy in the National Health Service', *Health Services Management Research*, 2 (1): 38-46.

Harrison S, Hunter, D. J., Marnoch, G. & Pollitt, C. (1991), 'General management in the NHS: the initial impact 1983-88', *Public Administration*, 69: 61-83.

Hearn, J. (1982), 'Notes on patriarchy, professionalisation and the semi-professions', *Sociology*, 16: 184-202.

Hood, C. (1991), 'A public management for all seasons?', *Public Administration*, 69: 3-19.

Houlihan, B. (1988), 'The professionalisation of public sector sport and leisure management', *Local Government Studies*, May/June: 69-82.

Johnson, T. (1972), *Professions and Power*, London, Macmillan.

Kouzes, J. & Mico, P. (1979), 'Domain theory: an introduction to organisational behaviour in human service organisations', *Journal of Applied Behavioural Science*, 15: 449-469.

Leach, S., Stewart, M., Davies, H. and Lambert, C. (1992), *Local Government: its Role and Function*, York, Joseph Rowntree Foundation.

Lipsky, M. (1980), Street Level Bureaucracy, New York: Russell Sage.

Major, J. (1989), *Public Service Management: the Revolution in Progress*, London: The Audit Commission.

Merton, R. K. (1968), *Social Theory and Social Practice,* New York: Free Press.

Millerson, G. (1964), *The Qualifying Associations: a Study in Professionalisation*, London, Routledge.

Morgan, G. (1990), *Organizations in Society*, London, Macmillan.

NHSTD (1991), *Bureaucracy to Enterprise*, London, NHS Training Directorate.

Nichol, D. (1990), NHS Management Executive News, December.

Nicholls, R. M. (1989), 'Central-local relationships in the aftermath of Griffiths, *Health Services Management Research*, 2(1): 58-63.

Normand, C. (1993), 'Changing patterns of care - the challenges for health care professions and professionals' in Malek, M., Vacani, P., Rasquinha, J. & Davey, P. (eds), *Managerial Issues in the Reformed NHS*, Chicester: Wiley.

Nutley, S. (1991), *Understanding change in the public sector: a local authority case study*, Unpublished PhD Thesis, University of Aston, Birmingham.

Olsen, .J .P (198,7) *The Modernisation of Public Administration in the Nordic Countries*, Bergen, University of Bergen.

Parsons, T. (1937), 'The Professions and Social Structure' *Social Forces*, 17: 457-67.

Parsons, T. (1951), 'Social Structure and Dynamic Process: the Case of Modern Medical Practice', in *The Social System*, Glencoe, Free Press.

Pollitt, C. (1990), *Managerialism and the Public Service*, Oxford, Basil Blackwell.

Poole, R. K. (1978), *The Local Government Service*, London, Allen & Unwin.

Raelin, J. A. (ed.), (1985), Special issue on 'The dilemma of autonomy vs control in the management of organisational professionals', *Human Resource Management*, 24(2).

Reed, M. & Anthony, P. (1992), 'Professionalising management and managing professionalisation: British management in the 1980s', *Journal of Management Studies*, 29: 591-613.

Roach Anleu, S. L. (1992), 'The professionalisation of social work? a case study of three organisational settings', *Sociology*, 26: 23-43.

Spybey, T. (1984), 'Traditional and professional frames of meaning in management', *Sociology*, 18: 550-562.

Stewart, J. (1990), 'Alternative futures for local government', address to RIPA's post annual general meeting, reported in *RIPA Report* 2(1): 3-5.

Stewart, J. (1993), *Accountability to the Public*, London: European Policy Forum.

Stewart, J. & Walsh, K. (1992), 'Change in the management of public services', *Public Administration*, 70: 499-518.

Stewart, R. & Smith, P. (1988), 'Lessons for managers', *The Health Service Journal*, 21st January: 90.

Strauss, A., Schatzman, L., Ehrlich, D., Bucher, R. & Sabshin, M. (1963), 'The hospital and its negotiated order', in Freidson, E. (ed.), *The Hospital in Modern Society*, New York: Macmillan .

Strong, P. & Robinson, J. (1990), *The NHS Under New Management*, Milton Keynes, Open University.

Torrington, D., Weightman, J. & Johns, K. (1989), *Effective Management*, London: Prentice Hall.

Wall, A. (1989), 'Griffiths five years on', *Health Services Management Research*, 2(1): 47-52.

Weber, M. (1919), Politik als beruf, published in English as 'Politics as a vocation' in Gerth, H. H. and Mills, C. W. (eds), *Max Weber: Essays in Sociology*, London, Routledge, 1948.

Wilding, P. (1982), *Professional Power and Social Welfare*, London, Routledge.

PART V

CONCLUSION

13 The future: Realism and diversity?

Ian Glover and John Leopold

Introduction

In this chapter we discuss the main arguments which have preceded it, relating them to some general issues and ideas about the future of NHS management. We start with a story which raises some broad issues. This story and the discussion of these issues may not at first seem very relevant to the main concerns of this book. However they are, as readers will see. Just as they help to contextualise NHS management, so they also help emphasize and explain its wider significance.

A Continental comparison

In the mid 1970s a prominent UK professor of engineering visited several Continental countries to see what he might usefully learn about engineering education. He departed as a sceptic, being firmly convinced of the high academic rigour of UK engineering science degree courses and very suspicious of the Continental notion of producing graduate engineers capable of making a strong practical contribution in industry shortly after taking up their first appointment.

He returned a year later with his views altered fundamentally, full of enthusiasm about the Continental, and particularly the German approach, to engineering education. He had learnt how Continental engineering students had received a broad secondary education, far broader than A levels, before entering university. At that stage students were generally able to speak three languages, and had taken a broad mixture of other arts, social science and science courses. The technical universities that they attended were as prestigious as any other kind, with engineering attracting at least its fair share of the most able numbers of each generation.

The structure of German engineering degrees (called diplomas, roughly equivalent to UK masters degree level in their intellectual demands) was very like that of UK medical degrees. Thus the first half, roughly of about three years of the course, was like the pre-clinical stage of a UK medical degree, and largely covered theory. The second three years roughly equated to the clinical part of a UK medical degree. It involved a considerable amount of practical project work, guided by 'engineer professors' with considerable industrial experience as well as high academic qualifications and achievements. The nature of this work, and of the theory and secondary education that had preceded it, ensured that the resultant Diploma Engineer (Diplom Ingenieur, in German) was not only a technical specialist who was also broadly educated, but also someone who understood well, the commercial, financial, human resource and corporate-strategic aspects of management, principally as they related to the industrial sector for which they had been educated.

In contrast, the typical British engineering graduate had studied the scientific theory relevant to his or her kind of engineering for three years. 'Management' or 'liberal studies' subjects tended to be tacked on to the main, 'real engineering' parts of the course. The notion of liberal studies being added on to 'humanise' the engineer was felt to be insulting by most students and by many engineering academics, too. Similarly, the 'topping up' of engineering courses with such management subjects as accountancy and marketing, seemed to assume that the management *of* engineering was superior to any management *in* it, and that management was, in general, a superior activity to engineering (Armstrong, 1996). Compared with their Continental counterparts, UK engineering students appeared to lack both self-confidence and the ability to communicate it to and to develop it in others. Unlike the former, they had generally not chosen to study engineering rather than science at university: they had been inadequately qualified to gain admission to science courses. Thus, engineering degree courses in the UK, while rigorous, tended to be second-best choices, 'mere applied science', which sheltered under the wing of 'pure' science. On the Continent, and again unlike the UK, such courses produced confident and fully-fledged practical and very well-educated engineers, not only with the potential, but fully expected to rise to the highest levels of their employing organizations. These tended, once again unlike their counterparts in the UK, to be engineer-dominated.

The professor returned to the UK, made his views known to his professional colleagues and discussed them with management researchers. He quickly came to realise that it was far more likely, in the UK, for business and management education to be expanded with the hope of improving UK industrial and general economic performance, than for engineering education to be made more attractive to the most able school leavers. After digesting this unpalatable conclusion, knowing that business and management education could never do much to help UK companies make better products, the professor turned his mind to finding a different way of improving the UK's economic performance relative to that of its main Continental competitors.

Eventually he stood his question on its head by asking how the UK might help to bring the latter's levels of performance down to UK levels. The answer came to him quickly: export pretentious and grandiose business and management courses to Germany and hope that sales are good. However attempts to make this happen since the mid-1970s have generally been very unsuccessful, even in France, a country with its own special grandiose traditions, although the joke has helped to sustain the professor's reputation for having a good sense of gallows humour.

This shaggy dog story is largely true, and relevant to this book's concerns in more ways than simply one of raising more doubts than those expressed so far about imposing general business management knowledge and practices upon complex specialist activities and expecting their performance to improve automatically. We know, for example, that while doctors in the UK may have long taken medical degrees which are organized along lines generally similar to those of Continental engineering education, and thus involve practical as well as theoretical learning, they have nonetheless mainly and long been taken by people with three A level GCE passes, people much narrower in a formal educational sense than their Continental counterparts. It is not surprising, therefore, that when UK doctors are compared with senior Continental engineers, the former are felt to be just as intelligent, but with more rough edges, slightly narrow but very able super-technicians, rather than cultured people who combine the best attributes of the specialist and the generalist.

The context of NHS management

In this book we use the NHS as a metaphor for the problems of UK management, especially regarding the relationships between professions and management, professionals and managers, professionalism and managerialism. In the other two books based on papers from the 1993 Stirling Conference on Professions and Management, we consider the problems of UK management and professions in a broad and general way in *The Professional-Managerial Class* (Glover and Hughes 1996a) and we consider the recent situations and experiences of a broad range of (non-medical) professions in *Professionals at Bay* (Glover and Hughes 1996b). What we are about to argue here, a major theme of these two books, is that management and the UK or Anglo-Saxon or Anglo-American management movement, have been deployed aggressively, in the forms of hyper-rationalization, hyper-differentiation and hyper-commodification, in the last twenty years or so in the UK, partly in order to make professions and professional work more efficient, effective and economic (the 'three Es' of some recent 'new wave management' thinking), less inward-looking, broader in scope, and more user-friendly.

In Glover's and Hughes' introduction to *The Professional-Managerial Class* the main distinguishing characteristics of UK management are spelt out. The points made include a number of significant Anglo-Continental comparisons, because, it is argued, the differences between Anglo-Saxon and Continental European assumptions and practices regarding education and training for work, the formation and status of occupations, the ways in which knowledge and skills are developed and used, and the most effective ways of dividing and managing labour, vary fundamentally, systematically and very revealingly in France and Germany and the countries that they influenced. These differences are summarised through a comparison between an Anglo-Saxon or Anglo-American 'Business Management' and a continental European 'Technik' set of assumptions and practices. There are five major areas of contrast between the two approaches. First, the Business Management approach emphasizes a relatively short term approach to economic effort and human development; a relatively passive economic role for government; rationally guided search behaviour and planning in organization and management; it valorizes consumption or some other end state or goal; and believes that a generalist with management qualifications should be able to manage anything (we call this 'management *of* '). The 'Technik' one, conversely, emphasizes a relatively long term approach to economic and human development; an active economic role for government; unpredictable ingenuity in organization and management; valorizes production and other socially useful processes; and believes that organizations and sectors should be run by specialists with deep experience of them (we call this 'management *in*').

One specifically important distinction between the two approaches consists of their ways of classifying and organizing subjects for study. In the Business Management countries the arts subjects include languages, literature, history, the fine and performing arts, religious subjects and some of the social sciences, with anthropology, business and management subjects and sociology, more likely to be classed as arts subjects, and economics, political science and psychology more likely to be classed as sciences. The 'sciences' include all of the physical and natural sciences, medicine, and engineering and technology - these often called 'applied science' - and the social sciences, indicated above. In the 'Technik' countries the classification scheme is much clearer. 'Kunst' subjects are the fine and performing, that is the 'doing', arts, such as writing novels, painting, acting and so on. They are taught in art colleges and their outputs are judged by aesthetic criteria. 'Wissenschaft' means science, or 'knowledgeship', or scholarship, all broadly defined, and the subjects that it includes are *all* those which are studied in order to discover the truth about and to increase understanding of relevant phenomena. All natural and physical and social sciences and religious subjects, languages, literature, history and geography, all belong, because all are concerned with the search for truth. They are taught in the traditional universities, and their outputs are judged in terms of truth or falsifiability, or rightness or accuracy against some agreed, predetermined, scale. Finally, there are the 'Technik' subjects. These are mainly taught in technical universities and other technical, commercial and administrative institutions. 'Technik' means engineering literally, although it has also been called 'our word technique with a capital 't' and a knighthood'. Its outputs are judged in terms of their practical utility, using such criteria as fitness for purpose and value for money. In this classificatory scheme, engineering is not 'mere' applied science, or even part of science at all. It is regarded as being at least as difficult, and probably of more social value, than science.

However the main Business Management versus 'Technik' distinctions that concern us here are those which identify three different kinds of senior, management-level, job holder. In the Business Management countries there are, first, *custodians*, mainly products of liberal arts and pure science courses in the traditional universities. They are normally employed for their 'trained minds' and for the 'helicopter quality' of being able to rise above detail, rather than for any specialist knowledge that they might have. They are (or were) expected to be able to occupy senior posts in almost any sector. It is (or was) assumed that they were broadly educated, mainly and simply by virtue of them having attended elite schools and universities, mixing with clever people studying a wide range of subjects. They have dominated the highest levels of the UK civil service for many years, and many other organizations which expect their top managers to display sophistication and social presence.

Second, and also in the Business Management countries, there are *professionals*. These tended to have provincial and less sophisticated backgrounds unlike the Cambridge-Oxford-London metropolitan ones of the custodians. Professionals tended to perform complicated and difficult specialist tasks like those of accountants, engineers, surveyors and market researchers, below the management levels at which custodians were employed. They have long made up the bulk and the core of the UK managerial stratum, although they have increasingly been graduates, either in their professional specialist or other subjects or both, and they have increasingly been elbowing custodians out (not literally!) of senior level posts. However in some sectors professionals have always been dominant: major examples include doctors in health care, lawyers in legal practices, academics in universities, clergy in churches, accountants in accountancy practices and management consultancies, surveyors in surveying practices, and engineers in engineering and design consultancies as well as in some but far from all industrial and cognate sectors. In general, but not in the church, the 'old' universities, and the senior levels of health care and the law, where they have long been and continue to be dominant, professionals tended to form a sort of provincially based 'second eleven' in UK management, although as noted above professionals and other invariably graduate, forms of expert labour, nowadays increasingly dominate all levels of it.

In the 'Technik' countries, the third type, *technocrats*, dominate all levels if not *at* all levels. We are using the word technocrat in a more ambitious way than the way in which it is usually understood in the Business Management countries. A Continental European technocrat, in our eyes, is a top job holder who is a (very) broadly (and deeply) educated specialist-cum-generalist. This is a correct use of the term technocrat because technocracy literally means rule by technically expert people. In the Business Management countries with their 'custodian' tendency to look down on the 'merely' technical, 'technocrat' is usually a slightly pejorative term used to describe, in the slightly memorable words of a former colleague, 'a nerd who has made it', or more precisely a relatively narrowly educated and/or trained specialist who exercises power in their employing organization. The sort of doctor-manager currently being developed through management education and training in the UK, in ways partly designed to overcome the relative narrowness of A levels and especially the lack of some aspects of management in medical education, is very close in many respects to 'our' kind of 'true', 'Technik' country, technocrat.

What we have largely seen, so far in this chapter, is the broad notion of the differences between the approaches to management, and so on, adopted in the 'Technik' countries and in Business Management ones, of which the UK is a significant example. These differences concern a given nation's whole approach to how people should work, and they are fundamental and influential and tell us a lot about the distinctive characteristics of UK management (Child et al., 1983; Glover, 1985, 1992; Hampden-Turner and Trompenaars, 1993). We must now ask what we should be looking for in considering what the book tells us about the ways in and the extent to which the NHS is a sort of metaphor for the problems of UK management.

The nature of NHS management

First, we should emphasize how, like any sector of employment in any society, the NHS is unique. To name but a few of its characteristics, it is in the public sector; exceptionally large in terms of its resources, activities and numbers employed; domestic not international in its operations; its tasks are infinitely varied, complex and difficult; its goals are unclear; it is subject to an exceptionally wide range of political and economic influences; and it is an organization uniquely and specially close to the hearts (metaphorically), minds and bodies (physically) of British people. It is run mainly by 'special' kinds of people too: dedicated, yet often ambitious, highly qualified and skilled, often bloody-minded and usually tough-minded, yet also caring and even tender.

At the same time, the managers and the managements of the NHS do have the five Business Management characteristics, tasks and patterns that are similar to many, faced by most other managers and management in the UK. First, they are required to determine or choose between priorities in order to cut costs. In the NHS such decisions can be exceptionally painful in every sense, and there is very often a strong element of short term expediency about them. The purchaser/provider split exacerbates this short termism by injecting unnecessary uncertainty into relationships and interfering with logical and stable approaches to resource allocation. Second, the role of the government in bringing about the managerial changes of the last twenty plus years has been quite firm overall, but day to day control of grassroots, even regional level, management has been almost entirely conspicuous by its absence until recent years. However, the NHSME now intervenes considerably in many aspects of NHS management. In spite of the rhetoric of empowerment and so on, directives emanate from it thick and fast.

Third, as most of the chapters, for example those by McNulty et al., Greenfield and Nayak, Bennett, Tilley, Dopson, FitzGerald, Ashburner, and Harrison and Nutley indicate, there is plenty of evidence to the effect that NHS management is guided, in general, by the Business Management philosophy's faith in rationally guided search behaviour, and there is also plenty of evidence, in the same and other chapters, for emphasizing the limitations of this approach. The two major limitations, are, first, the fact that health care is a useful art influenced by science (part of broadly defined 'Technik'), and in no realistic sense a science as such, and second, that only a few of the forces which influence the health of the public are subject to control by or influence from the NHS and government.

The fourth factor of the Business Management approach to running things, is that of emphasizing consumption or some other end state or goal over the process of achieving it. This is also apparent in the ways in which the NHS is managed, insofar as the practical effects of criticisms of the NHS's work are almost always directed at the supply side, the NHS's staff, rather than at the demand one (patients and other members of the public). This point is explained more fully below. The fifth and final feature, faith in and emphasis upon the value of the 'general' management *of*, rather than specialist management *in*, health care, is very apparent, and not in need of explanation.

We also feel that there is plenty of evidence, throughout most of this book, of processes of hyper-differentiation, hyper-rationalization and hyper-commodification. Since 1948, but most especially from 1974 onwards, the pace of organizational and managerially-induced change has generally accelerated. Attempts to bring growth and diversity (differentiation) under control (rationalization) *have* involved objectification of the 'products', health and illness and the care of healthy and ill people (commodification). This sort of 'postmodernization' process has arguably been a worldwide phenomenon, hardly unique to the NHS, the UK, or to the Business Management countries, although it may well be more apparent in all three of these than in most other sectors, other Business Management countries, and the 'Technik' ones.

The evolution of NHS management

How, and how effectively, have NHS professionals been resisting the encroaching forces of managerialism? And has part, an NHS part, of a professional-managerial class been growing up in the NHS, and is there evidence of a long-term trend towards the growth of some sort of health care technocracy? It is important for professionals to resist non-specialist, non-expert managerial domination, partly so as to maintain control over important skills and the development of them, partly so that the mixture between the strategic and the expert specialist aspects of management-level work remains at or near the optimum. Evidence of effective professional resistance to managerialist encroachment is not very apparent in the chapter by Bryson, Jackson and Leopold. In that instance NHS human resource managers appeared to be too weak to assert themselves, even in order to bring about changes desired by their superiors. However, most UK personnel or human resource managers have long occupied weak and ambiguous positions, and they are not a very significant or numerous group in the context of the issues under discussion (Legge, 1991).

The position of doctors is far more important in the NHS context. Regarding general practitioners, Greenfield and Nayak, in their chapter, suggested on the basis of their evidence that these types of doctor were likely to be very resistant to managerialism and commercialism, but very unsure, at least at first when confronted by them, as to how to implement their resistance. In considering the effects on doctors of market controls in the NHS, McNulty, Whittington and Whipp found that the use of market controls could both worsen and weaken, and improve and strengthen, in different ways, the practice standards and the political situations of doctors in NHS hospitals. Bennett, in her paper, showed how some doctors could, by showing entrepreneurial drive, enthusiasm and single-mindedness, use their professional characteristics of autonomy, status and collegiality to enhance as well as defend their positions. Tilley's evidence, also on hospital doctors in periods of organizational change, led him to emphasize the greater significance of medical intra professional power relations, compared with those between doctors and other health care employees, for influencing which medical specialists tended to 'win', and which to 'lose', when managerial 'reforms' were being implemented.

Clearly doctors, if not other professionals in the NHS, are, in many circumstances, capable of resisting managerial change effectively, on the balance of the research findings referred to so far. The notion of gains being exchanged for losses is also seen to be significant: there is usually, it would seem, at least some sort of price to be paid by a professional group when it enhances its position in a time of managerial change. The chapters by Dawson, Sherval and Mole, and Dopson add further support to this point. However, FitzGerald's is rather different. She portrays a rather complex and ambiguous situation, with clinicians becoming, over time, both more favourable towards the idea of becoming involved in management, and better educated and trained in order to do so. She also implies that clinicians are likely to be a good deal more competent judges of professional standards and performance than non-medical general managers: in the long run this could and should augur well for those who would like to see the majority of senior management jobs in the NHS filled by appropriately knowledgeable and skilled doctors, and with nurses and other NHS professionals filling many others.

Ashburner, in her chapter, effectively takes this sort of thinking further, as she suggests ways in which cooperative working relationships between doctors and general managers can be developed. She also argues that if doctors are to maintain or enhance their situations, they must be prepared to cooperate flexibly with doctors from other specialisms than their own. The arguments of Harrison and Nutley, in the chapter before this one, emphasize and contrast both the force of the managerialist and commercializing forces on doctors, and the strength and relative success of the latter's resistance. Harrison and Nutley also confirm the findings of other studies which had showed how general management had clearly weakened the authority of other professionals in the NHS apart from doctors, especially that of nurses. In the front line, and thus absolutely crucial in delivering health care, nurses had been challenged, oppressed and marginalized as far as the exercise of managerial power was concerned. There is however, need for further studies of the position of nurses and PAMs.

Causes for concern

Here there is a very important and paradoxical parallel with production management in manufacturing industry. Child et al. (1983) compared the organization of production in the UK and West Germany and showed how, in the former, management and professional groupings tended to hive off, define as a mere cost, intellectually and politically out-gun, and generally marginalize production management, whereas in West Germany, production was 'the whole company minus sales and finance', which did all technical development work, and which was seen as the source of virtually all wealth for the future. In the UK, with its laissez-faire stance towards the development of occupations, production and its management had been marginalized, not only because many university educated people had learnt to despise the idea of working in factories, but also because professional groups, which traditionally gave advice to and produced services for individual clients, not goods for innumerable anonymous customers, had both encouraged similar attitudes while muscling in, often in destructive competition with each other, in and around manufacturing establishments, much to the detriment of the latter.

Other critics of this situation had advocated strengthening the power of the manufacturing 'line' management, and weakening that of such 'staff' professionals as personnel managers, accountants, and of the specialist professional engineers and research and development staff who merely planned, at arms' length, the work of making things, while not deigning to be involved directly in it. However, this criticism had later been mis-applied in the public sector, for example in local government, the NHS and the universities, where professionals were employed to provide services to members of the public, and *thus largely were the line management* (cf. Glover and Currie, 1995, on universities, and Ackroyd, 1995, on local government). Thus to deploy managerialist forces and ideas to weaken the situations of such core line staff as nurses and doctors in the NHS, is to exacerbate the problem, not solve it. In a very real sense general management and the commercialism that came hard on its heels in the NHS *are*, or are major parts of, the problem.

Another rather startling parallel in this context is offered in a seminal paper by Ackroyd and Lawrenson (1996), who show how US management thinking and practices, inappropriately introduced in the 1950s into UK car and truck, railway engine and rolling stock, and aircraft manufacturing, involved the mis-organization, mismanagement, antagonization, and eventually the largely wholesale breaking up of skilled labour forces and managements which might well, had they been nurtured and developed along then existing lines, have been turned into world-beating examples of very highly flexible and very highly skilled specialization. The arguments of Ackroyd and Lawrenson, together with those of Child et al., tend to suggest that the NHS 'reforms' of the last quarter-century are seeking, in their rather blind ignorance, currently accelerated by the apparent insouciance of elements of the direction from the NHSME, to do to the NHS what inappropriate use of US-style (Fordist) mass production techniques and arms' length financial manipulation of companies did to swathes of UK industry since the Second World War.

Causes for optimism

Against this pessimism about the management of the NHS we may however set the possibility of the creation of a professional-managerial class of doctor-managers, of nascent technocrats for and in it. This is, at least in some respects, being encouraged by the working out of several aspects of the NHS 'reforms' and by growing use of increasingly relevant and sophisticated management courses, including ones at masters level, by doctors, and unfortunately to a much smaller extent, nurses. The healthy (no pun intended) scepticism of doctors towards management, noted by several contributors to this book, is probably as good a starting point as any for such a development. Also it is not unreasonable to suggest, to say the least, that the giving of direct responsibility for all or most aspects of the management of health care in the UK to doctors, nurses and other health care professionals is long overdue. What however is perhaps of most interest in the late twentieth century 'reforms' of NHS management is their very confused - in practical, moral and political terms - character. A very long and winding route was chosen for getting to a very simple destination. But will the NHSME block the road at the end of the journey?

The future: responsible citizenship and the health of the nation

The title of this chapter uses the words realism and diversity. Our choice of them is to do with the need to look at the NHS from every angle in order to understand it more completely, but also to understand that there are many diverse influences affecting the health of the nation, as well as NHS management. The future of the NHS, and by implication that of its management, is now considered briefly, as follows. The NHS, like most systems of health care in most countries, faces the problem that demand for care will always exceed the supply, simply because ill-health, which is almost inevitable in a person's life, is painful, and death, which certainly is, are feared. Both costs and expectations normally appear to be excessive, and always rising. Several forces as well as human physical frailty have brought this situation about. Thus doctors themselves have raised public expectations to unrealistic levels. And in some respects the gullible public has been expecting too much, seeking medical solutions for a range of such largely non-medical problems as job insecurity, conflict at home and work, difficult relationships in general, and natural ageing processes. Also medicine has, of course, often delivered or helped to deliver dramatic results, such as joint replacements, coronorary bypass operations, and greater life expectancy. So demand for what the NHS can, apparently, offer has increased markedly since it was founded.

To improve the provision of health care by the NHS the best general method would almost certainly consist of a swathe of relatively simple and straightforward improvements of a rational bureaucratic kind, principally involving more proactively careful use and development of resources by doctors and nurses, and other NHS professionals, and long term development of their practical managerial capabilities in such areas as accounting, budgeting, purchasing, human resource management, and marketing and public relations (for non-profit-making organizations). Instead, however, there is the purchaser/provider split, the use of quasi-markets, not real ones, partly because purchasers are in monopsony situations, and the strong rhetoric, about winners and losers and so on, of a self-consciously, avowedly 'hard' kind of capitalist management, one which probably has far stronger roots in the imagery associated with the Victorian writings of Charles Dickens and Friedrich Engels than in late twentieth century UK business. Most UK business managers do not, in our experience, work to overcharge and otherwise cheat customers, or to put their competitors out of business. Instead they rely much more on trust, understanding and competent work. And further, the main problems of the NHS are not on the supply side in any case: they lie on the demand side.

What is most likely to make the NHS more effective in the long term is for more citizens to be encouraged to, and themselves to, wean themselves off the notion that acute medicine can offer quick fixes for any unpleasant condition from acne or boredom to heart failure or cancer of the colon. Citizens should be educated to be more active in looking after their own health and to vote and campaign for policies on nutrition, exercise, expectant and nursing mothers, health education, housing and the physical environment in general. *The Patients Charter* (1992) emphasizes the rights of patients, in line with the view that they are 'customers' of the Service, whereas it would be far more sensible to put much more emphasis on their responsibilities to themselves and others and the environment, and to further and practice the notion of active citizens as people who work in partnership with their doctors and nurses to maintain, improve and otherwise care for their bodies and minds, and relevant aspects of the environment. Doctors and nurses should continue to be encouraged to work like 'reflective practitioners' (Schön, 1991) using appropriately open discussion with patients and treating the 'whole person' and not just the malfunctioning bits of her or him. 'Holistic medicine'

261

should be practised by everyone and be the norm, not an alternative.

Patients are not customers, incidentally, in anything but a very important but nonetheless secondary and minor sense. They are the throughputs of the system, very often changed by their dealings with it, and there is not in any case a seller involved in the relationship, and if no-one is selling anything, how can there be a customer? Patients are better thought of as 'users', but they are far more, too, than either that or customers. Society is the customer of the NHS, of course, with patients' employers or employees, friends and families also customers in a lower-order sort of way. But a free society is made up of sovereign and active citizens whose responsibilities and rights should be co-equal. Citizens as patients should neither be perpetually welfare-dependent malingerers ('dangling at the nipple of state maternalism', in the memorable if perhaps one-sided words of Barnett, 1986, p. 359), nor spoilt, immature, impatient and self-centred demanders of instant solutions, with little or no respect for achievement, experience or expertise, professional or otherwise.

Conclusion

This book has offered a solid and not insignificant body of evidence about some aspects of the recent state of NHS management, and a number of arguments about the ways and the context in which it has been developing. It needs to be read along with evidence on the experiences of patients and other interested citizens, nurses and other NHS professionals apart from doctors and other NHS employees including non-clinician managers, and on the economic, social, political and other consequences of recent and current NHS management. We do think that the book contains enough material and arguments to raise very serious doubts indeed about the sense of the naive modernist project of achieving good health for all through rational management and efficiency savings, and about the sense of much, although not all, recent and contemporary Anglo-Saxon management thinking and practice.

References

Ackroyd, S (1995), 'Professions, their Organisations and Change in Britain: Some Private and Public Sector Similarities and their Consequences', paper to ESRC Seminar, 'Professions in Late Modernity', University of Lancaster, 30 June 1994, and Mimeo, Department of Behaviour in Organisations, University of Lancaster, 1995.

Ackroyd, S. and Lawrenson, D. (1996), 'Manufacturing Decline and the Managerial Division of Labour in Britain', in Glover, I. and Hughes, M. (eds), *The Professional-Managerial Class: Contemporary British Management in the Pursuer Mode,* Avebury, Aldershot.

Armstrong, P. J. (1996), 'The Expunction of Process Expertise from British Management Education and Teaching Syllabi: An Historical Analysis', in Glover, I. and Hughes, M. (eds), *The Professional-Managerial Class*, Avebury, Aldershot.

Barnett, C. (1986), *The Audit of War*, Macmillan, London.

Child, J., Fores, M., Glover, I. and Lawrence, P. (1983), 'A Price to Pay? Professionalism and Work Organization in Britain and West Germany', *Sociology*, Vol. 17, pp. 63-78.

Department of Health (1992), *The Patients Charter: Raising the Standard,* HMSO, London.

Glover, I. A. (1985), 'How the West was Lost? Decline of Engineering and Manufacturing in Britain and the United States', *Higher Education Review*, Vol. 17, (3), pp. 3-34.

Glover, I. A. (1992), '"But westward look, the land is bright"? Reflections on what is to be learnt from British management education and practice', *Journal of Strategic Change*, Vol. 1, (6), Nov-Dec 1992, pp. 319-332.

Glover, I. A. and Currie, W. L. (1995), 'The Strangest Contradiction? Academic Dogs and Managerial Tails in UK Universities', Paper presented at the Second International Conference on Professions and Management, University of Stirling, August 1995.

Glover, I. and Hughes, M. (eds), (1996a), "British Management in the 'Pursuer Mode", in *The Professional-Managerial Class: Contemporary British Management in the Pursuer Mode*, Avebury, Aldershot.

Glover, I. and Hughes, M. (eds), (1996b), 'The Challenge to Professions' in *Professions at Bay: Control and Encouragement of Ingenuity in British Management,* Avebury, Aldershot.

Hampden-Turner, C. and Trompenaars, A. (1993), *The Seven Cultures of Capitalism*, Doubleday, New York.

Legge, K. (1991), 'Human resource management: a critical analysis', in Storey, J. (ed.), *New Perspectives in Human Resource Management,* Routledge, London.

Schön, D. (1991), *The Reflective Practitioner: How Professionals Think in Action*, Avebury, Aldershot.

Index

266